THE END OF MEDICINE

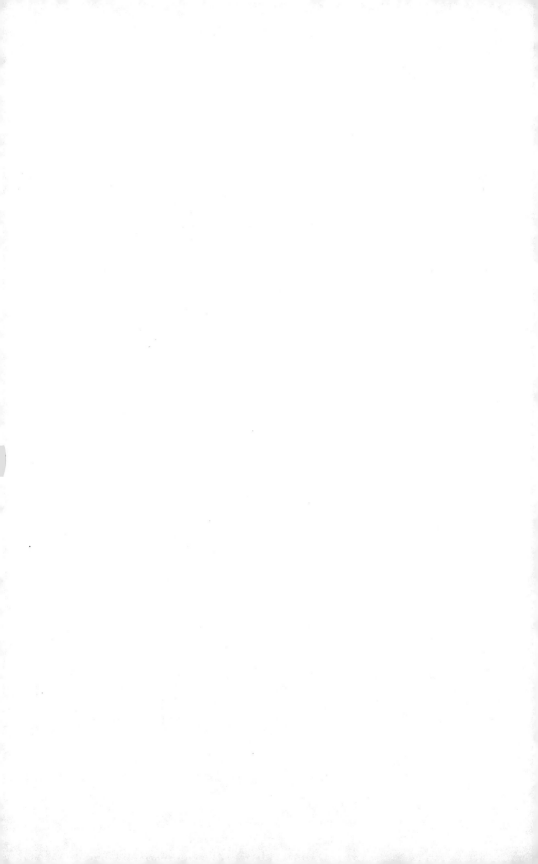

THE END OF MEDICINE

Kaare Bursell

Although in many instances the human body's response when adopting a
macrobiotic dietary practice is the resolution of most or all of our symptoms, no
guarantees are given that they in fact will. Furthermore, the disappearance of
symptoms does not mean the cause or causes have disappeared. It takes many years
of hard work, consistent practice and self-reflection to get through resolving the
symptoms of imbalance, some of which are resulting from ten, twenty, thirty or more
years of living out of balance. It is the individual's responsibility to work through
the ups and downs of the healing process and to keep learning and deepening our
understanding as we go. Your decisions are yours and are in fact the only valid
decisions for you.

This book was printed in the United States of America.

To order additional copies of this book, contact:
Xlibris Corporation
1-888-795-4274
www.Xlibris.com
Orders@Xlibris.com
53292

CONTENTS

"LIFE IS A WELL OF DELIGHT,
BUT TO HIM IN WHOM THE RUINED
STOMACH SPEAKETH,
THE FATHER OF AFFLICTION,
ALL WELLS ARE POISONED".

FRIEDRICH NIETZSCHE,
—THUS SPAKE ZARATHUSTRA.

ACKNOWLEDGEMENTS

This book is the second edition of the book originally published in April 2000, I have received the help and inspiration in one way or another from many people and I will mention some of them. They include my teachers Rudolf Steiner, George Ohsawa, Michio Kushi, and William Tims. Ronald Kotzsch, Ken and Ann Burns, Rod House, Bill Spear, Tanya Gagne, Tim Goodwin, Naboru Muramoto, Masanobu Fukuoka, Sherman Goldman, and Leonard Jacobs.

Also providing support and encouragement: Bruce and Marion Donehower, Aster Lazar, Roberto Marrochesi, Larry and Judy Cooper, Jean Baptiste Bello Mols Portu, David Briscoe, Carl Ferre, Al and Donna Wilson, David Jackson, William Thompson, Rodney Thomas, Bill Neall and Christina Derocher.

To Don Becket and Stephanie Kubicek, many thanks for proofreading and editing.

To my wife Patty and sons Alrik and Lief, my mother and father-in-law Pat and Smokey Lawrence, many thanks and of course to my mother and father, Ellen and Torsten Bursell.

To Madge and Francois Schelkens, who got me started on this wonderful journey.

To Bob Dylan and Neil Young, the two great troubadours of the times in which we live, for their wonderful music, inspiration and vision. To The Doors, who literally opened the door for me.

And finally, to the best teachers and inspirers I have been fortunate to meet, my students and counselees.

CHAPTER ONE

INTRODUCTION

This book describes how and why anyone can heal himself or herself of any non-congenital disease symptomology. This does not mean a guarantee is given and anyone undertaking to heal themselves using the methodology described herein must clearly understand they are solely responsible for healing themselves. This writing is based on over four decades of experience in the field of medicine, illness, health and healing and is offered on the basis of that experience.

Since the reader may be unfamiliar with a macrobiotic practice and the principles underlying it, an introduction is necessary. In recent decades it has become commonplace to talk about "curing" diseases in many and varied ways, including a macrobiotic practice. However, there has never been a cure for any illness, for in fact there is no cure for illness with the pursuit of finding a cure amounting to a colossal waste of time and money.

This is due to the fact that there is only one disease, accurately speaking, which is described as "living out of harmony, that is, out-of-balance, with the order of the universe." All illnesses manifesting any symptomology are an expression of the condition of being out-of-balance in our daily lives.

The phenomena of disease, illness and healing are thus deep and complex mysteries and for anyone to claim that a diet, procedure or medication of any description can cure or heal the body of being out-of-balance is sheer folly.

The folly stems from a complete lack of understanding of the constitution of the human organism in relation to the "order of the universe" and consequently what actually constitutes health, disease and illness.

It is helpful at this juncture, to undertake a meditation on the word health. The meditation begins with looking up the Old English root word for health and searching through the Oxford Dictionary of English Etymology for words with a similar root to the word health. This search produces the following additional words:

Welfare Whole Wealth Weal Home Hearth Heal Hale Earth Holy Heart Well.

The appropriate meaning of these words coherent with the intent of our enquiry, as given by the Oxford English Dictionary, is as follows:

> **Health**—soundness of body; that condition in which its functions are duly and efficiently discharged. Spiritual, moral, mental soundness or well being; salvation. Wholesomeness. Marked by intellectual soundness.
>
> **Heal**—to make whole or sound in bodily condition; to free from disease or ailment, to restore to health or soundness. To restore a person from some evil condition or affection (as sin, grief, despair, unwholesomeness, danger, destruction); to save, purify, cleanse.
>
> **Holy**—conformed to the will of God, entirely devoted to God; morally and spiritually unstained. Pertaining to God or the Divine Persons; having their origin or sanction from God, or partaking of Divine quality or character.
>
> **Hale**—free from infirmity; sound in constitution; robust, vigorous.
>
> **Heart**—mind in the widest sense, including functions of feeling, volition, intellect. The seat of feeling, understanding, thought. The depths of soul. The seat of love and affection. The innermost or central aspect of any process or thing.
>
> **Hearth**—that part of the floor or room on which the fire is made. (The modern version of the hearth is the kitchen and a separate fireplace).
>
> **Earth**—the ground on which we dwell, the abode of humanity.
>
> **Home**—the place of one's dwelling or nurturing, with the conditions, circumstances, and feelings, which naturally and properly attach to it, and are associated with it.
>
> **Whole**—in good condition; sound. Having all its parts or elements; having its complete or entire extent or magnitude; full, perfect, undivided; entire; unity.
>
> **Weal**—wealth, riches, well being, happiness, prosperity. The welfare of a country or community; the general good.
>
> **Wealth**—the condition of being happy and prosperous. Well-being. Spiritual well being. Thriving or successful progress in life, prosperity.

Welfare—The state or condition of doing or being well; good fortune, happiness, well being; thriving or successful progress in life, prosperity.

Well—sound in health, free from sickness and infirmity; of a character or quality to which no exception can be taken. In a good manner.

Health, rightly and comprehensively understood, lived and experienced, must include all the states of being with which this constellation of words resonate, individually, socially, economically and ecologically. It is not a mere matter of physical fact, and thus not to be confused with physical fitness in the athletic sense. The all-embracing vision of health must see it as a totality, expressive of a vigorous, abundant, creative tenor of life, the culture lived in such a manner, inclusive of the individual, family and society comprising this healthy culture, redolent with purity, honesty, compassion, and sublimity of feeling, intellect and spirit.

The intent of writing this small book is to describe a fairly simple home treatment, the ginger root compress, in the hope it will encourage its widespread use, along with a macrobiotic dietary practice. The main task is to explain why anyone may need to do a series of ginger compresses and how to know why you may need to do them.

The fundamental reason for embarking on a macrobiotic lifestyle is not to cure disease: rather it is to become a free and independent human being. In the effort required to so do a pre-requisite is we need to know how to take care of our physical body. Therefore I embed the description of doing the ginger compress regimen in the context of explaining disease, illness and health, as well as digestion and diagnosis.

If the reader is unfamiliar with a macrobiotic dietary practice, the contents of this book will serve as an introduction, However, if you decide to undertake the change to macrobiotic living, I do recommend you seek out people in your locality who are also living a macrobiotic way of life because much of macrobiotic thinking and theory is very different from conventional thinking and can be overwhelming to someone new to it.

Thus, any advice and information you can obtain from seasoned macrobiotic practitioners can be of help in avoiding various pitfalls and mistakes. The term macrobiotic practitioner is not limited to an individual who gives advice on a fee basis; it also means anyone who has been practicing a macrobiotic way of eating for several years.

In beginning a macrobiotic practice, I think it is critical to the efficaciousness of the dietary practice that a regimen of ginger compresses on the abdomen is also undertaken. Although the ginger compress is familiar to anyone who takes the time to read any of the macrobiotic books listed in the bibliography, it is a remarkable fact, at least to me, it is not done on a more widespread basis in macrobiotic practice. My personal experience of 32 years of macrobiotic practice and 23 years of counseling and teaching, has taught me it is immeasurably more difficult, if not impossible, for the body to undergo the healing process if one does not do the regimen of ginger compresses on the abdomen.

The reason this viewpoint is not widely held in the macrobiotic community, generally speaking, is, I believe, due to the remarkable improvement in bowel movement that most people experience soon after they begin a macrobiotic dietary practice. However, the fact that person has good, regular bowel movements does not mean that the bowels are not stagnated. This is the heart of the contents of this book, but in order to get to know how to do the ginger compress, it must first be understood how and why the intestines become stagnated, what "stagnation" signifies and how we can learn to recognize if our intestines are stagnated so we are sufficiently inspired to do the regimen of ginger compresses described later on in the book.

One further point. In the course of this book there are many references to yin-yang principles. Although there is a chapter on yin and yang later on, I must emphasize at the outset that the interpretation of yin and yang used in macrobiotic practice differs from the one used in Traditional Chinese Medicine today. The essential point about the two interpretations, which is very, very important to students and practitioners of Traditional Chinese Medicine, acupuncture, etc., to be clear about, is that the one in macrobiotic practice is not considered by macrobiotic teachers and practitioners to be the right, and the one used by Traditional Chinese Medicine the wrong, interpretation. The fact is, they are both correct in their interpretation; they can be used together if one understands them both, for they are based on entirely different perspectives.

CHAPTER TWO

THE DYNAMICS OF HEALING/ILLNESS

The first subject to focus on is the process of illness and the dynamics of food that underlies it, from the standpoint of the physical body[1]. The dynamics of food with respect to the dynamics of the human organism in terms of yin and yang[2] are illustrated in Figure 1. In the illustration those food groups, which lie at each end of what I call the Spectrum of Human Food, are considered to be extreme in terms of their yin and yang dynamics relative to the yin and yang dynamics of the human organism.

It will be observed that the food groups at each end of the spectrum are those that the majority of the world population consumes, especially in those countries that are technologically advanced. It will also be observed that all the technologically advanced countries are experiencing rapid and accelerating rates of degenerative illnesses[3]. as well as increasingly widespread incidences of infectious and parasitic illnesses. Concurrent these two phenomena is a gradual sense of modern medicine, for all its technological brilliance, being ill equipped to, and in fact lacks any realistic understanding of the causes of illness. Any methodology of treatment based on a lack of understanding of illnesses is necessarily an exercise in futility. As evidence, since 1960 the US and spent over 1 billion dollars a year on cancer research and modern medicine is no nearer to understanding cancer today that it was 45 years ago.

The question, which we should be asking ourselves, is how and why does illness come about and what does illness signify, since it is fairly clear the modern medicine has no idea. The reason why modern scientific medicine has no idea is because its epistemology (how it derives his knowledge) is based on the exhaustive investigations in physics and chemistry of inorganic matter, the world of materials—chemicals, minerals, rocks, soil, etc. Any knowledge derived from investigating the material world of inorganic lifeless matter is only pertinent when applied to inorganic, lifeless matter. If this knowledge is applied to living organisms of any kind it cannot hope to develop any understanding of living organisms.

Consequently, modern scientific medicine is epistemologically crippled in its attempt to understand clinical illnesses in human beings (as well as plants, insects, birds and animals). What is needed is an approach based on an epistemology that acknowledges living organisms are a different order of being than minerals, in order to begin to understand illness and how and why people become ill.

This epistemology has its antecedents in ancient traditional wisdom of both the East and West, which acknowledges that the fundamental basis of physical existence is spiritual. The spiritual reality of the human organism is it is actually constituted of two spiritual "bodies" in addition to the physical body. The physical body owes its appearance, growth, development and internal functions to what is variously called the etheric, life, formative or chi body, to which is attached the astral body, the basis of the soul. It is the soul that is the locus of feeling perception, cognition, memory, emotion, will, and so forth[4]

In this book, the human physical body is understood to be the visible manifestation of the dynamics of the life or chi body, where these dynamics are analyzed in terms of yin and yang. When we analyze the dynamics of the human physical body according to yin and yang, it is approximately 7 yin to 1 yang (the range of individuals is from 10 yin to 1 yang-5 yin to 1 yang). When we analyze the spectrum of human food according to yin and yang, the dynamics of the foods, which lie at the center the spectrum in Figure 1 (the underlined foods in the diagram), is also approximately 7 yin to 1 yang.

Figure 1.   **THE PROCESS OF ILLNESS/HEALING.**

7th Stage	"Return"
6th Stage	Cancer.
5th Stage	Chronic Toxemia.
4th Stage	Organ & Tissue Malfunction.

The Phase of Degeneration

3rd Stage	Accumulation.
2nd Stage	Skin Discharge.
1st Stage	Abnormal Discharges.

The Phase of Adjustment

YIN--YANG
Chemicals   Alcohol   Dairy/Nuts/Seeds   Seaweeds   Whole Grains   Chicken   Eggs
      Drugs   Spices   Fruit   Vegetables   Beans   Fish   Red Meat   Salt

---

16

If we ask why these particular groups of foods have a similar dynamic of yin and to the human physical organism, there are two hypotheses, which are not necessary mutually exclusive. The first, taken from the point of view of evolution, is a study of what has been a staple food for most of humanity

The answer is whole grains and vegetables. We can thus posit that, through the many centuries of eating a diet composed chiefly composed of whole grains and vegetables, the functions of the human organism have adapted themselves to optimum performance through eating these foods. Thus the Darwinian notion of "survival of the fittest" is amended to mean that, rather than those species are "fittest" which are stronger and more aggressive, they are those that "fit-in" the natural order as it has evolved over the millennia.

The second is that in the creation of the world and the human organism, the gods and spirits which have to do with the task of fitting the human organism to the world organism have created whole grains and vegetables as the most fitting food for the human organism.

And when we turn to native traditional wisdom we find plenty of evidence that our ancestors believed we, and the earth, have our origin in the spiritual worlds, and they thought the gods and spirits gave whole grains to humanity as a special gift.

There are many examples in sacred literature and I will cite only a few. In Chapter 1 of the Book of Genesis of the Bible is stated, "*And God said, behold I have given you every herb bearing seed, which is upon the face of the earth, and every tree, in which is the fruit of the tree yielding seed, to you it shall be for meat.*" [5] (Whole grains are unique among all plants in that they are the only plants which have both seed and fruit as one and the same entity.)

According to the Aztecs, Mayas and Zapotecs of Central America, man was made of corn. In the Popul Vuh, a sacred text of the Maya Quiche Indians of Guatemala, it states, "*Corn entered into the flesh of man. This was his blood, from this was the blood of man made.*" All across the face of the earth we find many native traditional ceremonies and seasonal rituals celebrating barley, corn, wheat, millet and rice.

As for the importance of food in human illness, according to the Taittiriya of the Upanishads, a sacred text of Ancient India, it is stated, "*Out of Brahman, who is Self, came ether; out of ether, air; out of air, fire; out of fire, water; out of water, earth; out of earth, vegetation; out of vegetation, food; out of food, the body of man. The body of man, composed of the essence of food, is the physical sheath of the Self. From food are born all creatures, which live upon food, and after death return to food. Food is the chief of all things. It is therefore said to be medicine for all diseases of the body*".

Hippocrates, the pre-Socratic Greek philosopher, who is widely considered the father of medicine in the West, and after whom the Hippocratic Oath of modern medicine is named, stated, "*Let thy food be thy medicine, and thy medicine be thy food*".

Thus it would appear the commonality of the yin and yang dynamics of the human life body (which is responsible for the dynamics of function of the internal organs and tissues of the physical body), with the yin and yang dynamics of a diet based on whole grains and vegetables means the physical organ and tissue functions will be vital and healthy if one eats a diet based primarily on whole grains and vegetables.

It also seems reasonable to posit a diet not based on whole grains and vegetables would likely result in organ and tissue illnesses and malfunctions. Today, in the developed countries of the world, especially so the United States, the diet is largely based on meat, sugar and synthetic, processed foods. In terms of the spectrum of human food, it is a diet in which the foods underlined in Figure 1 are largely absent. It must also be noted the abandonment of a whole grain and vegetable dietary practice is, in historical terms relatively recent[6].

The question arises, if the human organism functions vitally and healthily on a whole grains and vegetables dietary practice, how does it respond to a dietary practice based on meat and sugar, chemicals and refined, processed foods?

According to the principles of yin and yang (see Chapter 9.), if we eat a food, which is extremely yang, relative to the yin and yang dynamics of the human organism, we are necessarily attracted to food that is extremely yin; this we cannot help doing. Thus, if we eat meat, we have to eat refined sugar (or other extreme yin food like fruit and fruit juices, or refined flour products, or alcohol, or drugs like marijuana, cocaine, etc.),[7] since the greater the degree of difference between two opposite tendencies, the greater the force of attraction between them. When this combination of extreme yin and extreme yang is consumed on a regular basis, the body responds by increasing its rate of metabolism, which results in the generation of more waste metabolites than would otherwise be the case.

Now, we need to keep in mind that processes of the human organism functioning healthily and vitally with a dynamic of 7 yin: 1 yang. This means the organs of elimination function harmoniously with this dynamic of 7 yin: 1 yang, i.e., bowel movement, urination, exhalation, and skin breathing (all of which are technically termed "normal discharges" in macrobiotic terminology). Thus, the longer a person consumes these extreme foods on a daily basis, the increasing rate of metabolism generated leads to the eliminative organs become more stressed from having to process and eliminate the increasing flow of metabolic waste products.

In due course, it will become apparent to the person with this extreme pattern of eating that they are experiencing any or all of the following symptoms—difficulty with bowel movement, flatulence, skin perspiration, increasing frequency of urination, rapid and shallow breathing, bad breath and body odor. At some point in this process the organs of elimination begin to function improperly because they are becoming exhausted in their efforts to keep up with the excess production of waste metabolites. And the waste metabolites, which are toxic to the normal, healthy function of the cells and tissues of the body, begin to accumulate in the body. From this point on, and it really begins at conception (since most mothers today eat meat and sugar as their staple food), in most people, the integrity of the body is under siege, and the process of illness ensues as depicted in Figure 1. The hypothesis put forward here[8] is a description of the process of illness, which underlies all symptoms of illness, which have erroneously been identified as disease.

Disease, Healing and Illness.

A clarification is necessary here to specify what disease, healing and illness mean, as these are three distinct parameters. What is meant here is that disease is a fact of life and it cannot be prevented. Disease exists by virtue of the fact we live in a physical body and since we have no choice but to live in a physical body, we are necessarily subjected to the forces of disease.

However, all is not lost. We also have at our disposal the forces of healing, active in the etheric body. Our job then is to make sure we live in such a manner that we balance disease-inducing forces with forces of healing in our day-to-day lives. In the course of daily living the disease-inducing forces are continually oscillating with the healing forces. It is this relationship between the forces of healing with the disease-inducing forces that initiates the process of illness.

Therefore, we can say illness is the process whereby the human organism balances the forces of healing with the disease inducing forces. That is to say, illness is the process whereby the body heals itself. It is important to distinguish clearly these three separate yet intimately associated processes—that of disease, of healing and of illness.

Modern scientific medicine has gone to great lengths to record and has systematically tabulated all the symptoms (symptomologies) of illness human beings have thus far experienced. This is being done in the mistaken notion that illnesses are being described thereby whereas it has only succeeded in describing symptoms of the process of illness. There is only one process of illness, and all the symptoms of illnesses are indications of the stages or stage of the illness process a person is experiencing. For example, cancer is not an illness; it is one of the symptomologies of the process of illness as is arthritis, AIDS, influenza, etc.

The Stages of the Process of Illness/Healing.

The illustration (Figure 1.) is descriptive of the dynamic process of illness that is a response of human organism to a way living and eating which is extreme and out of balance with respect to the context of a human individual living on the earth. Since modern conventional life has little, if any, understanding of foods and their dynamics in terms of chi/ life forces, as we grow up we inherit a way of eating from our parents and the culture into which we are born. And little attention is paid to food other than assuaging our hunger, satisfying our appetite and pleasing our taste buds. Thus we are inattentive to and ignorant of what we are passing into our bodies, for the most part. The consequence of this ignorance (where we take the root of the word as meaning "to ignore") of all that we are putting into our bodies is depicted as the stages of illness in Figure 1.

Prologue.

The first stage of the process of illness is normal and healthy in regard to the functioning of the body, because the symptoms of abnormal discharge (they are called abnormal in distinction to normal everyday elimination of waste in the form of bowel movements, urination, breathing, skin breathing and physical and mental activity), such as fevers, headaches, and minor aches and pains, nasal discharges, coughing, sneezing, shivering, and, in more extreme instances, vomiting and diarrhea, are the outward visible signs of processes whereby the body is maintaining its internal physiological integrity, and at the same time, concrete confirmation of the integrity of the physiological processes whereby the body maintains its internal dynamic homeostasis.

The significant, world-shaking insight we can derive from the preceding, is the body demonstrates that it "knows" how to heal itself. The process of illness is, in fact, the way the body heals itself. That is, the symptoms of illness indicate the body is healing itself. Therefore the process of healing and the process of illness is one and the same process. Albeit, we have not yet penetrated the mysteries of disease, of healing or of illness, we can at least hypothesize the body inherently "knows" how to maintain its internal dynamic physiological integrity, and it is this integrity (which we can call the "wisdom of the body") which initiates the symptoms of illness, in order that the body maintains its integrity and viability.

I profoundly hope this idea is grasped with all the implications it entails, and the logical step taken to cease and desist in the developing and devising of expensive and ultimately futile methods to "cure" disease. For the line of thought we are following indicates that not only is there no cure for disease, (in the accepted usage of the word "cure"), it is not at least in the best interests of humanity that any cure for disease be found, if that were even possible.

After all, there are good and profoundly wise reasons why disease is present in the human experience. The whole problem of disease and its mysteries is a subject that requires another book. However, from what is presented here, you'll be able to work it out for yourselves. What is necessary to ask is the questions for ourselves—why is disease present in the world? what is illness signifying?, how does it develop?, what do my symptoms of illness mean for me?, and, what can I do about it?

In any case, what is almost universally meant by the notion of "curing disease" is fundamentally erroneous. The dictionary says "cure" means "to care for" so curing disease means to care for disease—actually what we are most interested is not to care for the disease, but to care for the person who has the illness.

And we can most propitiously care for the person who is ill by informing each other and ourselves about our illness, how and why we can heal ourselves and maintain our health, insofar as our present state of knowledge and wisdom allows.

The perspective here brought to bear on this problem is the present and continuing deterioration of the quality of life on the planet earth. Whether we are discussing economics, the environment, or social issues, all are fundamentally problems intimately bound up with the condition of the people who populate the earth—our physical, emotional, mental and spiritual condition. The continuing decline in the quality of the condition of the people in all these respects is fundamentally a problem of personal responsibility.

It cannot be overly stressed that the general trend of the past few decades has been the giving over of personal responsibility and personal decision-making to so-called "authorities" of one kind or another, whether they be corporations, governments, churches, universities, families, lawyers, doctors, etc.. As a result there has been a gradual accelerating decline in the ability of the individual to be free and independent. For all the talk and rhetoric and the resounding of the word freedom throughout the world, it remains a hope rather than reality.

It remains a hope because the bedrock of freedom is personal responsibility; we are the ones who are responsible for our lives; to point fingers and blame others for our problems means, for all practical purposes, we are abrogating our responsibility for personal freedom and independence. And the question of freedom has everything to do with and cannot be separated from our physical, emotional, mental, and spiritual health, keeping in mind the Meta—meanings of Health introduced in the previous chapter.

In regard of illness, people have gradually taken on the assumption when we get sick that there something wrong with us. We go to a doctor or some other health "expert" to "fix us up", which in actual fact can only be done by the individual concerned. This treatise is on how and why we may take personal responsibility for our physical, emotional, mental and spiritual condition. If the person reading this is relatively healthy, then this is the best time to start the manner of eating described here; if we are sick with some chronic infectious or degenerative illness, my experience of over 35 years of study, meditation, research and practice in the cosmos of healing, illness and disease tells me this is the best, most appropriate and sublime way of eating for our body in healing itself and maintaining its health.

Stage One.

What I want to focus on that this juncture is the dynamic of the process of illness/healing. Later I will address the physiological expression resulting from the dynamics described here. As already stated, referring to Figure 1, those foods lying outside the "area of balance" are extreme in terms of their dynamics of yin and yang relative to the yin and yang dynamics of the human organism. The hypothesis here is when foods of greatly differing polarities are introduced into the human organism, the strong reaction created between them leads to an acceleration of the dynamics of yin and yang of the life/etheric/chi body, causing an acceleration of the normal rate of the metabolic processes of the physical body.

As a result, the acceleration of the normal rate of metabolic processes means more production of waste metabolites than is the case in an individual whose pattern of eating is based more on those foods lying in the "area of balance". The longer a person eats those foods lying at the extreme ends of the spectrum of human food, then the more strain is put on the organs of elimination, as a result of the continuing excessive production of metabolic waste products.

At some point during this process the body begins to be unable to eliminate waste efficiently through the normal channels because the normal channels are becoming exhausted in their capacity to keep up with the excess production of waste (keeping in mind that the process of the normal functions of the eliminative organs is optimal—as well as the functioning of all the other organs and tissues of the body—when the body is nourished on a diet based on cooked whole grains and vegetables). The evidence that the organs of elimination are functioning at an accelerated pace in their attempt to keep up with the increasing production of waste is readily demonstrated by the rapid, shallow breathing, perspiration and body odor, bad breath, excessive bowel movements and/or constipation accompanied by flatulence, as well excessive urination, which is in fact the norm for most people today. As increasing production of bodily waste continues among people eating those foods lying at the extreme ends of the spectrum of human food, then these toxic waste products begin to accumulate in the body's fluids and tissues.

From the moment we begin eating meat and sugar, animal fats and chemicals, dairy food, refined, processed foods, etc., which in most cases is from the day we start our lives, the time comes sooner or later when the physiological integrity of the body is under siege and it responds by initiating the process of illness/healing.

The seven-stage process of illness/healing begins with the stage termed "abnormal discharges", initially described in the Prologue. I apologize to readers who have thoroughly understood what was said there; however as it states in the I Ching, "*it is through repetition that the student makes the material his own*".

Properly speaking, the body is always healing itself but these abnormal discharges are distinguished from the normal processes of elimination. Processes of abnormal discharge include fevers, sore throats, nasal discharges, coughing and sneezing, shivering, aches and pains, and in extreme cases diarrhea and vomiting.

The essential, critical point to understand is what these processes of "abnormal discharge" signify. They signify the actions undertaken by the body in restoring its internal, dynamic balance, in ridding itself of toxins. That is, these symptoms of abnormal discharge signify the body is healing itself, while the person is living a life, not only with respect to daily eating habits, but also in thinking habits, feeling, emotions, attitudes, morality, world view, work, relationships etc., which is a disorderly, out-of-balance, disharmonious, that is, dis-eased.

Herein lies the monumental error of modern scientific medicine[10]. It is indeed very difficult to describe how grotesque an error it is (in fact modern medicine amounts to a modern superstition) because of the manifold ramifications resulting in domains which are not usually connected with human, individual health, such as economics, the environment, social life (family violence, drugs, crime, etc.), politics, education and culture in general.

What has resulted is all the work, time, money and intent of modern scientific medicine is not devoted to solving the problem of illness or disease or healing but to solving the erroneous problem of treating the symptoms of the process of healing/illness. That is, all the hundreds of thousands of hours devoted by scientific medical researchers and professionals have been utilized in devising or finding ways to treat the symptoms of illness. Thus, all the talk about health care and health maintenance amounts to merely the treatment of the symptoms of illness and cost control regarding this, without paying attention to or even acknowledging the factors leading to the development of the symptoms of illness.

Modern medicine thinks the body is a machine, functioning like any other machine. As if our body is a car and one morning we get into it to go to work, we put the key in the ignition and the car will not start. Since we know nothing about the way the car works, we get a mechanic to look at it. He or she looks it over using diagnostic equipment and pronounces the starter defective. It is recommended we replace the defective starter with a new one, the job is done and, lo and behold, the car starts up immediately when we turn on the ignition, and off we go.

This is fine and sound when we are dealing with machines, but it is a grotesque error to approach the human body at the level of machines, as if it had all the functions and characteristics of a machine(albeit an elaborate and complex physico-chemical machine)[11]. However, a great deal rests on humanity extricating itself from this error, more than I can even begin to hint at here.

Immediately we begin to deal with the symptoms of illnesses as if they are the illness itself, any efforts, methods, procedures which are successful in treating the symptoms, e.g., the taking of pain killers to treat a headache, in reality only suppresses the symptoms of the illness being treated. This means our successful methods have resulted in developing procedures and methods that suppress the body's tendencies to heal itself. At the same time these methods are being administered, no attention is paid to the circumstances, the context, of a person's life leading to these expressions of the body's abnormal discharges; that is, the body healing itself.

We assume the purpose of medicine is to aid the body in asserting its functional integrity, (which is what it is demonstrating in manifesting the symptoms of discharge). However, what we see is modern medicine does the exact opposite. The injecting of synthetic drugs and chemicals into the body is merely administrating more powerful toxins for the body to eliminate. I note here over one hundred thousand people die every year as a result of taking medications, making death by pharmaceutical drugs the 5th leading cause of death in the United States[12]. Thus, it can be emphatically stated that if sick people recover after being administered various medications, it is testament to the remarkable recuperative and self-healing forces of the body that the person recovers, in spite of, rather than because of, the taking of the medication.

If it is true that medicine in its ideal form is to aid the individual in "curing"(that is, taking good care of) oneself, then modern scientific medicine is a degenerative, destructive medicine, actively promoting illness. To the very extent modern scientific medicine appears to be successful in devising methodologies to suppress the symptoms of illness in all its manifold forms, this means it is actually succeeding in promoting disease. In other words, modern medicine is itself a powerful disease-inducing force.

However, if we understand that any symptoms a person's body may be expressing indicate the person's body is not in balance with respect to the internal dynamics of yin and yang of their life or etheric body; and, furthermore they indicate the bodily processes which are undertaken by the body to restore its internal dynamic homeostasis to balance, then the proper medical approach is to let the symptoms run their course while endeavoring to address the causes why the body has become out-of-balance in the first place! In so doing, by simply adjusting the daily diet[13] to a proper balance in terms of yin and yang as indicated in Figure 1, the body is supported and aided in the process of recovering its functional integrity, and thus revitalizing and regenerating its internal functions, organs and tissues.

A formidable obstacle to this idea is the hubris of modern scientific medicine and the idolatry people evoke towards it. It is widely considered that modern scientific medicine is the apogee of medicine, the most advanced and sophisticated so far in the history of humanity. However, this notion is far from being true and it will not to be too long from now that we will look back at modern scientific medicine as being thoroughly antiquated, an aberration in the annals of medicine.

Nonetheless, today people regard modern scientific medicine with awe, and at the first symptoms of abnormal discharges, mistakenly believing something is wrong with their body, they go to a doctor or pharmacy to obtain a medication to make the symptoms go away. In this case, since no attention is paid to the context, including diet, as these symptoms are occurring, nothing is done to change the context itself.

As a result, American people (this is also true of the people living in any modern developed country) have been experiencing for several decades now, and will continue to experience in increasing numbers as long as people continue to live in the way we do, massive plagues of manifold degenerative and chronic infectious illnesses, faced with which modern scientific medicine is not merely helpless, it is also one of the chief protagonists of these plagues.

I must say that I do not mean modern scientific medicine has done this consciously; it has gradually occurred generally speaking, unwittingly, unconsciously over the past 100-200 years. This actually makes it all the more puzzling and mysterious, that a medicine that has as its tenet: the Hippocratic Oath, an oath taken by all modern physicians, as follows (after Hippocrates, the ancient Greek generally regarded as the father of Western Medicine):

I SWEAR in the presence of the Almighty and before my family, my teachers and my peers that according to my ability and judgment I will keep this Oath and Stipulation.

TO RECKON all who have taught me this art equally dear to me as my parents and in the same spirit and dedication to impart knowledge of the art of medicine to others. I will continue with diligence to keep abreast of advances in medicine. I will treat without exception all who seek my ministrations, so long as the treatment of others is not compromised thereby, and I will seek the counsel of particularly skilled physicians where indicated for the benefit of my patient.

I WILL FOLLOW that method of treatment that according to my ability and judgment, I consider for the benefit of my patient and abstain from whatever is harmful or mischievous. I will neither prescribe nor administer a lethal dose of medicine to any patient even if asked nor counsel any such thing nor perform the utmost respect for every human life from fertilization to natural death and reject abortion that deliberately takes a unique human life.

WITH PURITY, HOLINESS AND BENEFICENCE I will pass my life and practice my art. Except for the prudent correction of an imminent danger, I will neither treat any patient nor carry out any research on any human being without the valid informed consent of the subject or the appropriate legal protector thereof, understanding that research must have as its purpose the furtherance of the health of that individual. Into whatever patient setting I enter, I will go for the benefit of the sick and will abstain from every voluntary act of mischief or corruption and further from the seduction of any patient.

WHATEVER IN CONNECTION with my professional practice or not in connection with it I may see or hear in the lives of my patients which ought not be spoken abroad, I will not divulge, reckoning that all such should be kept secret.

WHILE I CONTINUE to keep this Oath unviolated may it be granted to me to enjoy life and the practice of the art and science of medicine with the blessing of the Almighty and respected by my peers and society, but should I trespass and violate this Oath, may the reverse by my lot.

Especially when the main tenet of his medicine, "Let thy food be thy medicine and thy medicine be thy food" has degenerated to the extent that modern scientific medicine is fundamentally harmful to the human organism.

In the first stage of the illness/ healing process, at the first signs of symptoms, many of us run to get the medication for cold, fever, headache etc. Then, if we recover—which we usually do, since our illness/healing process is only in its initial phase—we do not change anything in our lives, least of all our dietary habits and so stage two develops.

Stage Two.

This stage is signified by, in addition to the previous symptoms of abnormal discharge, the discharging of toxins through the skin. These are so-called skin diseases and there are hundreds of them, including psoriasis, impetigo, athlete's foot, eczema, dandruff, acne, pimples, rashes, etc. The important point to understand is that skin diseases signify the organs of elimination—the kidneys, lungs and large intestine—are becoming clogged with excess toxins, fats and animal proteins. Thus, local applications may be helpful in ameliorating some of the discomfort of the skin conditions, but they are fundamentally useless with regard to resolving the conditions themselves. Instead, the systemic imbalances of these organs must be changed by changing our daily eating habits.

At this stage the body still has enough of a reservoir of vitality to bring the toxins to the surface of the skin; but at some point, sooner or later, in the process of illness/healing the inherent vitality of the body begins to weaken and become run down from the constant effort of pushing the toxins through the skin, in addition to the symptoms manifesting in stage one, and gradually toxins begin to build up in the body's organs and tissues.

Stage Three.

The accumulation of toxins internally signifies this stage. Here occurs the silent development of cysts, abscesses, fatty deposits, fibrous deposits, calcified matter, papillomas, etc., in the organs and tissues of the body. Usually these depositions are occurring without the knowledge of the person, other than becoming overweight, at least with regard to physical symptoms.

The way of knowing that these accumulations are occurring is that they are evoked psychologically. In addition to yin and yang, an important conceptual tool lying at the foundation of a macrobiotic practice is the Five Transformation Theory. Although it does not lie within the scope of this book to go into a detailed explanation of the theory, it does have an important application here.

One of the important aspects of the theory is that when any of the organs of the body begins to become burdened with excess toxic buildup, this affects the quality of the etheric or chi activity of the body, which is the basis of the structure, function, growth and development of the organs and tissues. The disturbances thus engendered in the dynamics of the chi or etheric forces permeate into the soul activity in the person, thereby leading to mental, emotional, and spiritual disturbances. As Rudolph Steiner stated *"All psychological disturbances have their origin in the disturbances of the physical body; all physical disturbances have their origin in disturbances of the psyche, (soul)".*

As the accumulating toxins build up in the physical organs they affect or elicit emotional disturbances, which, in the Five Transformation Theory, are correlated with the organs. For example, if the kidneys/bladder become toxic or stagnated, the person so affected begins to feel anxious, begins to lose confidence and his troubled by fear. In the case of the lungs/large intestine, we become sad, morose and depressed. In the case of the spleen—pancreas /stomach, we feel worried and doubtful. In the case of the liver/gall bladder, we become frustrated, impatient, irritable and angry. In the case of the heart/small intestine, we become nervous, excitable and hysterical.

The emotional disturbances are of a chronic nature, and at least from the perspective of the person who is experiencing them, of "uncertain etiology". That is to say the person experiencing them is quite unaware of their origins.

It is important we not make the error of supposing that once we start eating a macrobiotically balanced diet and our organs begin to be cleaned and rejuvenated, then all our emotional problems will disappear like magic. We also have to address psychological disturbances by means of the psyche, that is, by meditation and self-reflection.

The first three stages of the symptomology of the illness process are referred to as the Phase of Adjustment and if no changes are made to alter the context of the person's life, then the Phase of Degeneration begins. The beginning of the phase of degeneration of the process of illness is the Fourth Stage.

Stage Four.

Here the accumulation of toxins in various organs and tissues leads to the dysfunction and malfunction of these organs and tissues, and eventually they become debilitated and unable to function properly. It is at this stage that heart disease, liver disease, kidney dysfunction, diabetes, diverticulosis, eye problems, asthma. etc., become evident. Currently there are over 2700 different disease syndromes recognized by modern scientific medical research.

Stage Five.

One of the major organs of the body, which is not normally considered an organ, is the blood. The blood stream has in the past been referred to as the "river of life" and functions as the great mediator of the activity of the organs and tissues of body. Here at the 5th stage of the symptomology of the process of illness/healing the blood itself becomes heavily polluted with toxins. In the previous two stages the blood has been depositing the toxic waste metabolites in the organs and tissues as a result of the inability of the eliminative organs to eliminate them. Here, however, the increase in the level of toxins has reached the point where the blood can no longer keep itself relatively clean and we reach the stage of chronic blood toxemia, which means long-standing poisoning of the blood.

In the symptomology of the illness/healing process, we know we have reached this stage by the body manifesting symptoms of chronic infectious illnesses, including, for example, hepatitis, herpes, syphilis, polio, tuberculosis, candidiasis, and the host of other chronic infectious illnesses, which are erroneously attributed to the organisms that give their names to the illnesses, e.g., salmonellosis, streptococcus, trichosomiasis, etc. The understanding here is that the infectious organisms presented in the symptoms are just one aspect of the symptomology of the 5th stage of the process of illness/healing, and are not the primary cause of the symptoms.

Of course, the Germ Theory of illness has long been a dogma of modern scientific medicine, but it is fundamentally erroneous, and in my experience, based on unsound and inattentive observation and illogical thinking.

In the history of modern scientific medicine and the Germ Theory, three individuals stand out as playing a role in its development. Two of them were French scientists, Claude Bernard (1813-78), a physiologist, and Louis Pasteur (1822-95), a chemist and bacteriologist. They had what can be considered an epic spiritual battle over the problem of the cause of illness.

Bernard took the position described here, with the condition of the body being the main, significant, principle to understand in the problem of illness, and the germ, if one is involved, being secondary. He made an analogy, where he said the relationship of the human organism to the microbe (the infectious organism, be it a virus, bacteria, spirochete, worm, etc.) is analogous to the soil in relationship to the seed that is planted in the soil.

Whether or not the seed (microbe) takes hold, germinates and flourishes in the soil (body), depends on whether the condition of the soil (body) is suitable for the germination and growth of the seed (microbe). Therefore, he said, all our scientific investigations must be directed to understanding how the condition of the body develops so as to make it possible for the germ to enter in, take hold and flourish there.

Louis Pasteur, on the other hand, maintained that the only significant factor in the development of illness is the microbe, and all our scientific investigations must be directed to studying and understanding the microbe, so we can eradicate it, and therefore solve the problem of illness. He believed that the microbe was the sole cause of illness. However, on his deathbed, Pasteur made an abrupt about-face, saying, in terms of Bernard's analogy, the soil is everything, the microbe only secondary.

Pasteur's story is similar to another major individual involved in the development of the Germ Theory of Disease, Rudolph Virchow (1829-1902), a German pathologist, anthropologist and political leader. He said on his deathbed that if he had his life to live over again, all his scientific investigations would be devoted to demonstrating germs attack already diseased flesh, they do not cause disease.

The history of modern scientific medicine is one in which the germ theory has held sway, and all scientific investigations have been devoted to developing pharmaceuticals, be they anthelmintics, vaccines and predominantly antibiotics, to treat the symptoms of the process of illness. This has led to many problems, and raised questions, the most significant of which is why is there a complete lack of understanding of illness or health or disease by modern scientific medicine.

The injection or ingestion of pharmaceutical medication of any kind into the human organism merely introduces substances which, in the case of antibiotics, are not only poisonous to bacteria, they also poisonous to the human organism. In fact, all pharmaceuticals are poisons for the body. These poisonous substances have in turn lead the to the human organism becoming even more intoxicated and, therefore, diseased.

What we need to ask ourselves is what is the role microbes—the worms, viruses, bacteria, and other parasites—play in the scheme of things. Among their many activities is they gravitate to dead and decaying organic matter, in both plants and animals and human beings, consuming the decaying matter and in so doing, makes such matter available as nutrients to enrich the soil and fertilize plant growth. Thus we can hypothesize that when the human organism is host to pathogenic organisms, this indicates the internal tissues and organs of the body are both dead and decaying.

I present a graphic illustration, which occurred a couple of years ago. I went out one morning to my backyard and I saw a dead mouse on the grass. I went over to take a closer look and the mouse carcass was swarming with ants. Now, no one in his right mind would conclude the ants were responsible for killing the mouse and devouring it. No, the mouse had died from some other cause, and the ants were devouring it and thereby cleaning up the carcass. So it is with microbes inside the organism—they gravitate to a diseased organ or tissue in order to clean it up while flourishing in the organ or tissue.

The fact that transmission of the organism can occur from a person hosting an infectious organism into another person, who then begins to show symptoms of carrying the same organism, merely means the second person's body is also in a state of decay, a suitable environment in which the microbe can grow and flourish, i.e., show evidence of pathogenic behavior. If a person with a healthy body comes into contact, whether by breathing, kissing or sexual intimacy, with the person who is hosting a microbe showing evidence of pathogenic behavior in their body—that is, they have herpes, hepatitis, AIDS, etc., or that they have eaten food that has E.Coli, or Salmonella—then on gaining entrance to the healthy body, the microbe will find the healthy body an unsuitable environment for its growth and replication, and either be destroyed by the healthy body, or simply die, and be excreted.[14]

Thus, the absolutely critical point to understand is microorganisms, worms, etc., are not the causative factors in infectious, or any other, illness; they are merely one of the symptoms. To put it another way, if the person has been diagnosed with, for example, pneumonia, and the sputum they are coughing up is cultured and is found to be riddled with a bacterium, say Pneumoccus, it does not follow the Pneumococcus is the cause of their pneumonia; the bacteria is simply one of the presenting symptoms of that person's pneumonia. It should also be pointed out that a person can have pneumonia or any other illness, without any microorganisms, worms etc., being presented in the symptomology.

We can then make the statement—pathogenic organisms are not pathogenic because they cause pathological changes in the organs and tissues; they are pathogenic because they are attracted to and flourish in organs/tissues which are undergoing pathological deterioration.

If a person has not died through the first five stages of the process of illness (keeping in mind that every stage of the process of illness is at one the same time the body attempting to heal itself under the imbalanced conditions in which the person is living), then we come to the 6th stage.

Stage Six.

Here the blood, in its attempts to maintain the viability of the physical organism, deposits the excess toxins in special sites, which I refer to as "toxic waste disposal sites", normally referred to as tumors, that is, cancer. We can imagine in the course of the illness/healing process in the Phase of Degeneration is the development by the body of an internal waste disposal process as the normal eliminative functions (external) become gradually exhausted and worn down in their capacity to eliminate toxins through the normal avenues of urination, bowel movement, exhalation and skin breathing. I do not intend to go into a long discussion on cancer except to say it is the last attempt by the body to maintain its viability under long-standing conditions over many years, even decades, including diet, that is out-of-balance. The only salient point is we can say cancer is an illness symptom which is redolent of everything that is out-of-balance in this culture. Cancer is overwhelming evidence modern civilization is entirely dis-eased in every area of human endeavor—eating, living, thinking, feeling, business, economics, medicine, education, politics, environment, etc.

. The statistics of cancer are astounding. The cancer rate, defined as the ratio of the US population who can expect to get cancer if they live to be 60 years old, was, in 1960, one in 16. In 1985, it was one in three; today, it probably approaches one of every two people[15].

Stage Seven.

I call the 7th stage of the process of illness "return" because in the I Ching—The Book of Change, it states *"all movement takes place in six stages, and the seventh brings return."* The term is taken in this context to mean that we return to the state we are in prior to birth, conventionally called death, or we take in hand our sick condition, acknowledge we are sick people living in a sick society, and recognize our sick condition is the result of our own mistakes, errors of thought, word and deed, and proceed to correct them, beginning with the dietary changes discussed, and so "return" to healthy life and living[16].

NOTES.

1. This is to alert the reader to the fact our dietary habits are not the only possible cause of illness.
2. It lies outside the scope of his book to explain how, analyzing foods using yin and yang arrives at this arrangement. The arrangement is a general one and, within each food group some foods are more yin and some foods are more yang relative to one another. I must also point out that the descriptions of yin and yang here are at variance with those of Traditional Chinese Medicine. This does not mean that macrobiotic practitioners consider Traditional Chinese Medicine to be in error in its interpretation. Suffice it to say the macrobiotic interpretation of yin and yang is based on a geocentric perspective, that of Traditional Chinese Medicine from a metaphysical one. As long as one is consistent in their interpretation and does not get them mixed up then errors will not occur.
3. For example, in 1960 the cancer rate in the US population, defined as the ratio people in the country who would get a cancer if they live to be 60 years old was 1:16. In 1985 it was 1:3. The illness treatment (erroneously called health care) costs of the US were 185 billion dollars in 1982, 750 billion dollars in 1991, 900 billion dollars in 1992 and exceed 1 trillion dollars in 1996. These costs surpassed 2 Trillion dollars in 2006.
4. For a detailed account of the complexities of the constitution of the human organism, see "Theosophy" by Rudolph Steiner (Anthroposophical Press, New York, 1971).
5. Authorized King James Version, verse 29.
6. For example, refined sugar intake in the United States in 1904 was four pounds per person per year; in 1985, it was 125 pounds per person per year.
7. Here lies the dynamic basis of drug use and abuse. That is to say, our physical addictions or desires have their origin in the attraction to consuming extremely yin substances, which is elicited when we eat meat or any animal protein on a regular basis. If we adopt a macrobiotic dietary practice, it is relatively easy to give up drugs and other extreme foods, drink and substances, as I can personally attest. On other hand, for any person trying to give up these substances without giving up meat, this is extraordinarily difficult.
8. I should point out this is a hypothesis for the scientific community; in the macrobiotic community, it is theory. The distinction is that a theory is widely accepted as a reasonable explanation of verifiable experience, whereas a hypothesis is an explanation put forward to be tested and if it is verified, it becomes a theory.
9. It must be emphasized that the "wisdom of the body" cannot be construed to reside in the physical body itself; that is, it has nothing to do with the laws of

physics and chemistry, which only operate in the domain of matter, outside the body. Rather, it resides in the dynamics of the life, or chi body, which is expressed in the dynamics of the physiology of the human organism.

10. It is important to make a distinction between modern scientific surgery and modern scientific medicine. The former is impressive in his ability to perform corrective and reparative work on broken bones, torn ligaments, bullet wounds, serious injury etc. On the other hand, modern scientific medicine, for all its advanced technology, and diagnostic procedures, cannot ever hope to lead to an understanding of illness or disease or health.

11. It is of interest to note how many prominent people in society think the human organism is a machine; just recently, and this was a surprising to me, I read Bill Moyers says he thinks the body is a machine.

12. *Prescription for Disaster* by Thomas Jay More, Simon & Shuster, 1998.

13. Feelings and emotions, attitudes, world view, relationships, work life, lifestyle etc. have also to be taking into account in terms of restoring balance but these aspects lie outside the purview of this book.

14. It is important to note when the body has successfully dispatched a potentially pathogenic organism, it shows evidence of having done so by having antibodies to that organism present in the blood. Thus, the presence of antibodies in the blood means the body has successfully dispatched the organism involved.

15. Putting cancer in perspective, in the United States, a person died of cancer every 56.8 seconds, which amounts to 564,740 people in 1996 (see Times Special Issue, The Frontiers of Medicine, Fall 1996, Page 20); in 1994 526, 000 people died, once every 60 seconds. AIDS, in contrast—up until 1992, 500, 000 people have died as a result of AIDS worldwide in a decade.

16. A note on AIDS, Acquired Immune Deficiency Syndrome. From the perspective of the dynamics of the symptomology of the process of illness, it appears to be a concatenation of the illness process in the one syndrome, which is an interesting observation. From what was said about the six stages of the dynamics of the process of illness, the human immunodeficiency virus, or any other virus does not cause AIDS. The scientific medical research community is belatedly beginning to catch onto this reality (long held by a virologist. Dr Peter Duesberg, University of California, Berkeley), as was reported the September 26, 1991 issue of Nature.

AIDS is a syndrome characterized as acquisition of functional deficiency of the immune system. So a line of inquiry to understand it is futile if it is maintained it is caused by a virus, the HIV, or any other microorganism. It is more accurate to say the presence of the virus indicates the deficiency of the immune functions of the body.

As for the etiology of the virus, it's as proposed here (with due respect to Michio Kushi as the first person who came up with this idea, at least to my knowledge, and to a program on mitochondria I saw on BBC television in 1975), that the decay or deficiency of the immune system, which is comprised of the spleen, kidneys, liver, white blood cells/lymphatic system and additionally, and, in my view, most importantly, the large intestine, is such that the internal environment of these organs have become so weakened through increasing toxicity that the normal organelles of a healthy cell of any one or more of these organs degenerate, and the process of degeneration is their devolution to primitive organisms, for example, viruses.

We can readily understand, from the description of the process of illness, these organs become damaged and toxic after many years of eating a diet based on meat, sugar, eggs, chemicals, and refined, processed foods as well as taking antibiotics and recreational drugs, alcohol etc. to the point the normal functions of immunity are compromised and the symptomology of AIDS develops.

CHAPTER THREE

DIGESTION

Introduction.

In order to understand the approach being taken here it is helpful to amplify more on what was said earlier on the constitution of the human organism. The physical body is understood to be a manifestation of the dynamic activity of the etheric/chi body, which is necessarily invisible to the physical sense organs. It is utterly impossible to understand the functioning of the human physical body if it is thought that it's functioning is according to the laws of physics and chemistry operating in matter. The fact that most people, including scientific medical researchers and workers, consider the human body to be an elaborate expression of physico-chemical activity is tragic and to be lamented because it is, strictly speaking, scientifically untenable[1], and has lead modern medical science to a complete, absurd, dead end. The shallow, hackneyed thinking of modern scientific medical researchers can hardly be better exemplified than in the statement by a scientific writer trying to explain why molecules evolve when he writes "molecules evolved because they have evolved to evolve"[2]. This statement sums up the futility of understanding living organisms by way of the epistemology of modern materialistic science.

The reality of the physical body is that it is the manifestation of the dynamics of the etheric/chi body. If the human body were only constituted of the physical and the etheric bodies then it would be a plant, for a plant is constituted only of the physical and the etheric bodies. However, the human being also feels, thinks, has memories and dreams, imagines and plans, and the body in which these activities take place is called the astral body. The relationship of these three, the physical, etheric and astral bodies, is such that if the human being were the only constituted of them, we would behave like animals.

In addition to these three the human being is also endowed with an ego or the "I"—which is what gives us our individuality. The key distinction to make between animals and human beings is that that in the case of any animal, once we understand the patterns of behavior of an individual of the species, we will know the behavior of all individuals of the same species. This is not the case with the human being (ideally!).

Digestion.

The process of digestion can be outlined as being comprised of the following activities:

Conscious activities.

Selection, preparation, cooking and serving of food and chewing the food when we eat it.

Unconscious activities.

Digestion—mouth, stomach, pancreas, gall bladder, duodenum, small intestine.
Assimilation (transformation)—small intestine.
Metabolism (anabolism and catabolism)—liver, spleen, pancreas, kidneys.
Elimination—large intestine, lungs, kidneys, liver and skin.

Our level of consciousness plays the most significant role in digestion because it is according to it that we involve ourselves in the selection preparation, cooking, serving and chewing of food.

Food is the basis of our physical existence. This is **not** the same thing as saying that food is the origin of our physical existence as human beings; or "we are what we eat" but, once having incarnated in a physical body, then it is our physical body which is our habitation for the duration of our life on earth. The physical body is the central, physical fact of our existence on earth, the vehicle for feeling, thinking and doing, which are all spiritual in origin.

Since the source of the substances with which we clothe our body every day is our daily food, it is not surprising food is of momentous significance to us. Although no one would deny that food is a subject that occupies our thoughts every day, there can hardly be a time in the history humanity when there has been less understanding of food than there is today. This is hardly surprising because the tragedy of modern materialistic science is that although it is singularly occupied with analyzing and studying the material world, and never before in history have more individuals been involved in this pursuit, there we will look in vain for any real understanding of the material world at all.

The world of nature surrounding us is the provider of the food we eat off of our plates (no matter how much as has been devitalized and refined in its passage from the soil to the supermarket shelf), and the fundamental source of our food is the plant world. We may take plants directly from the soil to be cooked and eaten, or we can eat them in the form of animal flesh, as well as animal milk in various forms. There's an abundance of choice, the key being—how do we know what to choose to eat?

Once we have made our selection, we prepare, cook, serve and eat the food, chewing it thoroughly before swallowing. It is up until the moment the food passes down our throat, if we are at all conscious of what we are doing, (the general level of consciousness of what we are eating is very low today); that we are in fact conscious of what we are eating.

These are the levels of consciousness (after George Ohsawa):

Supreme.
Religious—moral.
Social.
Intellectual.
Sentimental.
Sensory.
Mechanical.

When we apply these to the way we are eating, the mechanical level is where we are singularly, exclusively concerned with the mere satisfying of our hunger—this level is characterized as the "Hungry Beast".

At the sensory level, in addition to satisfying our appetite, we are particularly concerned with the taste of the food. The vast majority of present-day humanity is to be found at this level of consciousness of eating (as an all pervasive slogan of a few years ago testifies, "it's a great time for the great taste . . . .").

At the sentimental (emotional) level our preoccupation with food, in addition to satisfying the previous two levels, is to eat dishes we find emotionally satisfying; that is to say, we like food we grew up with, our mother's cooking, or we eat to give us a sense of comfort from the trials and tribulations of the day, or to fill our emotional emptiness, or to suppress our negative feelings.

At the intellectual level the main concern is whether we are getting enough calories, vitamins, minerals, etc.

At the social level we're concerned with eating the food of our ethnic heritage (Italian, French, Mexican, Chinese, etc.), or we are concerned with the social, economic and ecological consequences of our eating habits.

At the religion—moral level we eat in order to support our religious and spiritual development.

At the supreme level we eat whatever we like without it unduly affecting us in any way. It is important to know that these levels are not separate from one another, as we develop our level of consciousness, each level of our consciousness of eating is built upon the previous levels of consciousness of eating, so the appropriate way of eating of a fully integrated human being includes all seven levels of consciousness at the same time.

And once the chewed food has passed into the esophagus, we are only vaguely aware of what transpires as it passes into the stomach, and then only if something untoward happens during the passage. As the food we have chewed and ingested settles into our stomach, we are only aware of what is happening there in a dream-like state of consciousness. When the food enters the small intestine we are utterly unconscious of what is taking place there.

Digestion itself is actually completed by the time the food enters the body of the small intestine. The process of digestion is itself unique to each individual person on a day-to day basis. The digestive process actually functions in this way; imagine one takes the tongue and pulls it from the tip down through the body so that it is inverted and elongated—thus we have the digestive system, with the inner mucus epithelial lining of the intestinal tract being a modified taste organ. As the chewed[3], and digested food enters into the esophagus, stomach, etc., the epithelial lining "tastes" the food, and according to what it tastes it secretes the appropriate amounts of the appropriate digestive substances, such as enzymes, acids etc. The organs which secrete digestive substances are the salivary glands, the mouth, the lining of the stomach, the pancreas, the gall bladder, and the lining of the duodenum and esophagus.

Digestion accomplishes the breakdown of the solid food to a finely emulsified homogeneous fluid called chyme. The chyme also consists of water, undigested material such as roughage (fiber) as well as bacteria, which also play a significant role in the digestive process. In terms of yin and yang, the formed, solid (more yang) food becomes more yin during the digestive process. Thus the food is ready for assimilation.

This scenario being developed here makes it clear that the most significant organs in the onset and development of the process of illness are the organs of digestion, assimilation, metabolism and elimination.

After twenty-five years of counseling thousands of people from all walks of life and of every hue of skin and ethnicity, and from observing, using facial diagnosis, people on the street, in restaurants, on the bus and train, on television, and in newspapers and magazines, I have found that one organ condition is present in everyone, without exception.

This is the long-standing stagnation and depletion of function and increasing build-up of toxic substances in the large intestine. I propose the large intestine is the hub of the elimination process and, by extension, the process of illness. The condition of the large intestine not only determines the function of the large intestine itself, it also determines how the kidneys, bladder, lungs, liver and skin function. We can look at the relationships of these organs from various perspectives to arrive at an understanding of the dynamics of their mutual functional inter-relationships.

Figure 1.

THE FIVE TRANSFORMATIONS.

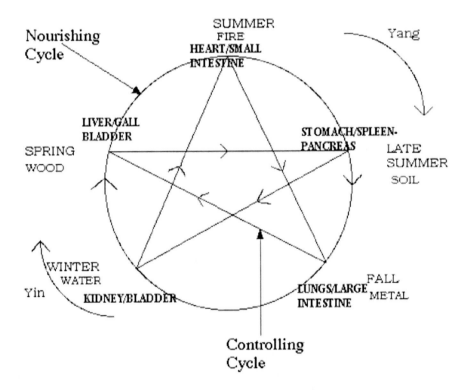

One of the more useful concepts for studying these relationships is the Five Transformations Theory. The diagram (see Figure 1) shows the relationships of the organs of the body according to the theory. These relations are the dynamics of the etheric/chi forces that flow between the organs, with the outer cycle been the "Nourishing/Mother-Son" relationship, the inner one being the "Controlling" relationship.

It is important to have a true picture of the relationship of the etheric/chi body to the physical body. Let us take a walk in the woods where we find a beautiful, sparkling lively stream making its way through the trees and shrubs. We observe the stream and see the water flowing downstream, and in the water we see evidence of various currents manifesting their activity by the ripples, eddies, waves and turbulences in the stream.

Thus we can say the stream is constituted of the water and the currents flowing in the water. In this picture of the human body, the etheric body is analogous to the currents flowing in the water, and the physical body is analogous to the water in which the currents are flowing.

Now imagine we have not visited the beautiful stream in the woods for many years and, in the time since our last visit, a factory with housing for the workers has been built upstream from place we first encountered the stream.

When we return to the same spot we now see the stream is filled with all the effluent of the activities of the factory and the people living there. To our dismay it is now toxic with oils, tar and chemicals and the detritus of waste. The water is now filled with all this material and we find where there was once a beautiful sparkling dynamic stream is now dark and muddy, flowing sluggishly, smells, and is stagnant and noxious.

This is a picture of what happens to the human body when toxic stagnated matter builds up the tissues and organs of the body and necessarily, consequently, the activity of the etheric body also becomes sluggish and stagnated.

Study of the Five Transformation Theory[4] shows us that if and when the large intestine and small intestine become infiltrated with toxic accumulations, this will cause their etheric/chi flows to become stagnated, and this stagnant chi flow will effect stagnation of the function of the lungs, heart/small intestine, kidneys/bladder, and liver/gall bladder.

Furthermore, according to the theory, the tissue of the body that is a manifestation of the Metal stage of transformation is the skin. Thus the condition of the skin is directly related to the condition of the lungs/large intestine; its condition being the outward manifestation of the condition of the lungs and large intestines.

In the case of the small intestine, according to the theory, its condition will affect the condition of the heart, stomach/spleen—pancreas, lungs/ large intestine as well as the blood vessels.

In the context of the elimination of waste metabolites generated by the activity of body cells, the organs responsible for regulating and controlling this are the large intestine/lungs, kidneys/bladder, liver/gall bladder and the skin. Our study of the Five Transformation Theory makes clear the relationship of the large intestines to the other organs of elimination. However, the very nature of the theory is that all the organs are important and they all influence each other in various ways. It does not emphasize the importance of the large or small intestine over any other organ. Thus we needed another perspective in order see why the intestines are particularly significant, more so than any other organ, in the onset of illness and recovery of health.

The perspective that points to this is to look at the processes of the human being as analogous to the growth of a plant (see Figure 2.). The essential point to grasp is that the small intestine/large intestine are the fulcrum from which the whole human being lives, in that they are the roots of the body from the perspective of providing the means whereby assimilation of nourishment and elimination of waste is the basis of the physical sustenance of the human organism.

If we return to the picture of the physical body as being the outward manifestation of the dynamics of the etheric body, we can say the food we eat and digest on a daily basis is "taken up" by the etheric body and "molded" into the organs and tissues of the body, and the etheric forces also imbue the organs and tissues with their particular activities and functions. It is important to understand that the physical food which is taken in by the organism is in and of itself dead matter, and if it were the case that the human body was nothing but matter, it could not exist, for in that case it would indeed be a handful of dust.

Figure 2.

THE HUMAN ORGANISM AS A "TREE".

7. SEED	"WORKS"
6. FRUIT	SELF-DEVELOPMENT.
5. FLOWER	SPIRITUAL/EMOTIONAL/MENTAL CONDITION.
4. LEAF	CELL (ORGANS)
3. BRANCH	HORMONAL/AUTONOMIC NERVOUS SYSTEM
2. STEM (SAP)	BLOOD
1. ROOTS	INTESTINES

SOIL (of Growth and Development)   FOOD AND THINKING

It is not an exaggeration to say this perspective points to the determinative role the condition of the small and large intestines play in our lives, the physical as well as emotional/psychological aspects of our life. As the diagram shows, the condition of the "roots" of the body determines the condition of the blood (the "stem/sap" of the body), and the blood in turn crucially influences the condition of the "leaves", (the cells of the organs and tissues of the body, the physical organism). Just how crucial will be shown in the next chapter.

Since the physical organism is permeated with the etheric body, to which is "attached" the soul or astral body, it is readily understandable how the condition of the physical organism permeates into the astral body via the etheric body, thereby influencing our mental, emotional and spiritual condition, the "flower" of our growth.

The fruit of all this is what I call ""self development" by which I mean the development or lack thereof, of moral character, self-knowledge, wisdom and understanding of life. By "works", I mean those efforts of our life on earth we are leaving for future generations, in the form of poetry, paintings, inventions, buildings, writings, or, on a more personal level, how we influenced and transformed our community, family, children, peers, friends, enemies, and so forth.

It is necessary to point out this growth of the "plant" of the human being is not a uni-directional flow; each of the phases of growth influences all the other "stages", so that, to cite only one example, the "flower" does indeed influence the "root". Thus when I discuss healing, this means not only do we have to change our way eating and change the condition of our intestines, we also have to address our way of thinking, attitudes, world-view, and our spiritual life. These will be addressed in the chapter on Macrobiotic Healing.

Fig. 3.

ANATOMICAL ARRANGEMENT OF LARGE
AND SMALL INTESTINES- HEALTHY PERSON

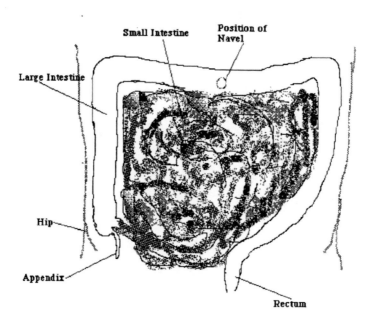

The above diagram (see Figure 3.) is a rendition of the small intestinal anatomical arrangements in relationship to the large intestine in the healthy human organism. This perspective shows us the large intestine surrounding the small intestine, like a pair of hands joined at the wrists delicately holding a flower arrangement. It points to the insight that the quality of flow of etheric forces in the large intestine influences the quality of flow of the etheric activity of the small intestine, and therefore its functioning.

Another perspective that can help us to understand the critical role of the small and large intestine is shown in Figure 4. This schematic outlined depicts the single "organ" of the mucous epithelial lining of the digestive tract (mouth, oral cavity, throat, esophagus, stomach, duodenum, small intestine, large intestine, rectum, anus) and the respiratory tract (nose, sinuses, trachea, upper bronchi, alveoli) becoming the skin, the external epithelial lining. It is this "organ" which encloses the body with a protective barrier, which is also the interface of our relationship with the physical world around us. If we look at it with an artistic, imaginative eye (granted, I am not much of an artist!), the mucous epithelial lining of the intestines is the "center of gravity" of this arrangement. Thus we can surmise that the condition of the mucous epithelial lining of the intestines will have ramifications in all areas of the mucous epithelial lining and, furthermore, the condition of the mucous epithelial lining will have ramifications for all the organs related to the mucous epithelial lining.

Fig. 4.

THE "BOUNDARY ORGAN" OF
SKIN(EXTERNAL) AND MUCOUS EPITHELIAL
LINING(INTERNAL).

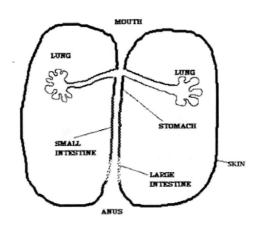

What is the function of the mucous epithelial lining? Its functions are manifold and I will focus only on a few here. The mucous epithelial lining is composed of mucus cells, and among their functions is they secrete various substances into the "lumen" or cavity bounded by them. These include substances to aid digestion, various antiseptics and lubricants, which are contained in the mucus.

In the healthy human organism mucus is always being secreted as a necessary lubricant, moisturizer and antiseptic, and is generally clear and somewhat watery. However, in the case described in the first two chapters where an individual's dietary habits are based on the food groups lying at the extreme yin and yang ends of the spectrum of human food, and the lifestyle habits are also imbalanced, then the extreme dynamics in terms of yin and yang of these foods entering the body induce an increased rate of metabolism.

The increased rates of cellular metabolism means more toxic waste products of tissue metabolism enter into the bloodstream; more, that is, than is the case of someone consuming a diet based on the foods lying in the center of the spectrum of human food according to yin and yang. In the case of an individual eating foods lying at the extremes of the spectrum, the organs of elimination, for reasons explained in the previous two chapters, cannot eliminate the consequent increase of toxic waste efficiently. In this case the mucous epithelial cells begin to secrete copious amounts of thick, viscous, discolored, mucus in order to remove the excess production of toxic waste metabolites generated by the extreme way of eating.

In other words, excessive production of this thick, sticky mucus is the means by which the body gets rid of excess toxins as the organs of elimination gradually become exhausted in their ability to accomplish this process efficiently. The consequence of this will be explored in the next chapter.

NOTES

1. I want to point out that the word science comes from the Latin "scire." which means, "to know". Of course, there are many ways of knowing, with modern materialistic science being only one; to assert that modern materialistic science is the only way of knowing the truth about any phenomenon is therefore patently untrue, unacceptable and unscientific.
2. K. Eric Drexler, in his book "Engines of Creation—the Coming Era of Nanotechnology."
3. It is important to chew our food well. A helpful technique I learned from David Jackson, to ensure and train ourselves to thoroughly chew our food is, once we have placed the food in our mouth, begin chewing while we place our utensil on the plate, fold our hands together, and count our breathing for five inhalations/exhalations before we swallow and take another mouthful.
4. The chapter on the Five Transformation Theory in "Healing Ourselves" by Naboru Muramoto (Avon Books 1973), is a useful starting point for study, as well as the section "Healing With The Seasons" on my website—see the chapter "Getting Started" for the URL.

CHAPTER FOUR

BLOOD ALCHEMY

In this chapter I will first give a description of the macrobiotic theory of assimilation of nourishment, as it occurs in the healthy human organism. Then will follow a description of the process of the assimilation of nourishment in an unhealthy human organism.

Assimilation.

The small intestine is the organ responsible for assimilation of nourishment into the human organism. It occupies a large volume of the pelvic cavity, a highly convoluted tube beginning where the duodenum becomes the jejunum, approximately 4-5 inches from the left side of the body, under the last rib bone. From here it twists and turns to become the ileum[1], which terminates some 25-30 feet later at the ileo-cecal valve, the junction of the small and large intestines, approximately 2 inches in from the right hip bone.

Figure 1. is a diagrammatic representation of a transverse section of the wall of the small intestine. It reveals five distinct players, beginning with the outer serous lining, then the longitudinal muscle, then the circular muscle, then the sub mucous and mucous layers. The latter two exhibit circular folds projecting into the lumen of the small intestine, thereby increasing its internal surface area, which is further vastly increased by the millions of fine, motile, finger-like projections, about one millimeter in length, the villi, lining the wall of the small intestine[2].

According to macrobiotic theory the villus is the focal point of the assimilation of nourishment. The theory proposes the villi are the active players in the assimilation of digested food substances, where the process of assimilation is the transformation of these food substances, initiated by the villi and completed by the liver, into the red blood cell (erythrocyte).

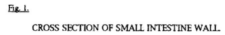

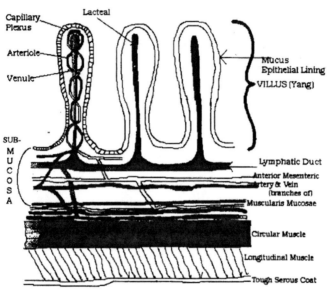

Fig. 1.

CROSS SECTION OF SMALL INTESTINE WALL.

The basis of the theory of assimilation as the transformation of food into blood is yin-yang theory. According to yin-yang theory, where in this description the more yang tendency of etheric/chi dynamics is given by the symbol (Δ) and more yin is given the symbol (V), the process is as follows:

In the process of digestion the solid (Δ), formed (Δ) food is broken down to liquid chyme (V), moving from the upper body (V) to the center of the body (Δ), in a downward direction (Δ). Further, the soft (V), hollow (V), long (V) and more undulating (V) structure of the small intestine signifies its more yang (Δ) function.

Additionally, we must always keep in mind the spiritual foundations of existence, including the physical body. In the case of the intestines, both small and large, the spiritual foundation is called the "Hara", where in oriental medicine Hara is referred to as the "Sea of Chi" or the "Ocean of Infinite Ki", where "chi" is the Chinese, and "ki" is the Japanese word for etheric forces According to the Five Transformations Theory, the small intestine is perceived as being the yin manifestation of Fire, the most highly charged "plasmic" form of chi.

The villi projecting toward the center the lumen of the small intestine indicate they are more yang (Δ), which is further demonstrated by their constant motile activity (Δ). Thus, according to yin-yang theory, the more yang etheric movement of the villi attracts the more yin etheric activity of the chyme, and due to the highly charged chi of the small intestine, a sparking of mutual attraction occurs at the tips of the villi. Somewhat analogous to, but an inverse image of, a sparkplug igniting fuel in an enclosed chamber.

In this description, the homogeneous (**V**), differentiated (**V**), liquid (**V**) chyme is gathered in (Δ) by the villus (Δ) and transformed into a discrete (Δ), bounded (Δ) cell (Δ), while simultaneously the mucous cells (Δ) are secreting mucus (**V**) into the lumen of the small intestine.

This momentous event continues as a discrete cell (Δ), being the transformation of chyme, called the "*monera*"[3], is extruded into the capillary plexus/lacteal nexus of the villus. The monera are more yin cells relative to the red blood cell; they go through a process of transformation in several stages of the white blood cells, from the more yin neutrophil, through basophil, monocyte and lymphocyte, all of which contain a nucleus, to the most yang cell, the erythrocyte or red blood cell, which is anucleated, that is, the nucleus is extruded during the transformation from the lymphocyte. Theoretically this process begins in the capillary plexus of the small intestine and is completed in the liver. In the lacteal and the lymph systems a white blood cell remains a white blood cell, see Figure 2.

<u>Fig. 2.</u>

SUMMARY OF TRANSFORMATION OF FOOD INTO BLOOD.

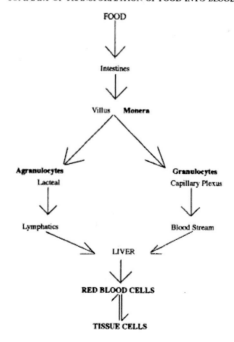

FOOD

Intestines

Villus   **Monera**

Agranulocytes   **Granulocytes**
Lacteal   Capillary Plexus

Lymphatics   Blood Stream

LIVER

RED BLOOD CELLS

TISSUE CELLS

The granulocytes are white blood cells containing small granules in their cytoplasm, namely the neutrophil, basophil and eosinophil, and the agranulocytes are those containing no granules in their cytoplasm, being the lymphocyte and monocyte.

The red blood cell or erythrocyte can be seen as the "master cell" of the body, while the monera is the "mother cell" of the body. The red blood cell, in addition to playing crucial roles in metabolism, respiration and in the body's defense activity, is, according to macrobiotic theory, capable of transformation into a cell of any organ or tissue of the body according to the body's needs at any particular moment. The reason for its capacity for transformation is the red blood cell is extraordinarily flexible due to it being informed by both strong yin and yang tendencies, which it therefore manifests. The flexibility of the red blood cell is demonstrated by its structure, the shape of the cell being indented toward the center and bulging towards the periphery. Moreover, it also shows the ability to take on any shape as it squeezes through tight spots in the capillaries, being a "bag" that can be formed into almost any shape. The normal red blood cell contains small amounts of material relative to the thickness of its outer membrane, which means that any radical change of shape does not stretch the outer membrane to the extent of rupturing it, as would be the case with other cells.

In summarizing, the process of digestion is food becoming chyme, and the process of assimilation is chyme being transformed into red blood cells. In terms of yin and yang, digestion is the yinnization of food into the highly differentiated homogeneous liquid of simple substances (plus fibrous material and other material the small intestine does not assimilate) followed by the yangization of chyme into the red blood cell. The red blood cell, because of its inherent dynamic flexibility, can be transformed into any organ or tissue cell of the body[4].

The theory of why the red blood cell can change into any organ or tissue cell is based on the knowledge that the physical organism is the physical "mask" or "mineral gesture" of the etheric body. It is the etheric body, which gives the human organism its particular form or shape, is responsible for the growth and development of the body, as well as for the form and function of the organs and tissues of the body, and their co-coordinated activity. Thus, every physical organ and tissue has its spiritual "mason", which gives the cells of the organs and tissues their particular form, arrangement, and dynamic of function. As a red blood cell makes its way out of the capillary into the etheric "field" or matrix of the organ or tissue, it is transformed by the etheric matrix of the organ or tissue into the cell of the organ or tissue in question, be it spleen, heart, nerve, muscle etc..

When the tissue or organ cells have undergone their cycle of activity, they are then extruded into the bloodstream, thereby transformed back into red blood cells, which are recognized by the spleen as being old red blood cells. The spleen macerates these old red blood cells and the resulting waste material is eliminated via the gall bladder as bilirubin, in the bile fluid secreted into the intestinal tract. It is bilirubin which is responsible for proper fat digestion and coloring the stools in our bowel movement.

This process of digestion and assimilation as the transformation of food into red blood cells is, overall, more yang, as the transformation of food into red blood cells suggests. There is also more yin process of assimilation, which is occurring simultaneously.

Before I describe that process, however, it is necessary to remind you the above description is the predominant way that digestion and assimilation occurs in the healthy human organism. The question arises: what happens in the process of the human organism becoming toxic and ill?

In the previous chapters it was stated the most people living on the earth today eat a diet consisting primarily of meat, eggs, refined sugar, potatoes, tomatoes, milk, fruits, chemicalized, frozen, refined, and processed foods, and it was described how this dietary habit leads to the secretion of copious amounts of thick, sticky mucus by the mucous epithelial cells lining the digestive and respiratory tracts.

In the case of the small intestine, this build-up of mucus eventually leads to a thick layer overlying and covering the villi of the small intestines, gradually building up inside the lumen of both large and small intestines. Of course, the food we are eating every day continues to pass through the intestines, and since the lumen is narrowing in diameter over the course of time, due to the build-up of mucus—the process I am describing takes several years, even decades, to unfold; the time it takes will vary according to individual circumstances. There comes a time when the food substances are having to squeeze themselves through this continuing narrowing aperture, and in doing so create pressure against the mucus build up. As time goes on, eating the normal daily diet, the increasing pressure causes the development of a thick, sticky, dense layer of mucus up against the mucous epithelial lining, its density taking on that of a tar-like substance.

When this state is reached, the mucus being secreted by the mucous epithelial cells is effectively dammed up, and instead of going into the lumen, it backs up into the actual cellular tissue of the intestine, both small and large, into the sub mucus and muscle layers. It is this process of buildup of toxic waste material in the intestinal walls which I called Chronic Intestinal Stagnation. Figures 3. and 4. show examples of what happens to the gross anatomy of the small and large intestines, which have chronic intestinal stagnation.

Fig. 3.

ARRANGEMENT OF SMALL AND LARGE INTESTINE
AFTER SEVERAL YEARS OF EATING THE "meat and
sugar" DIET.

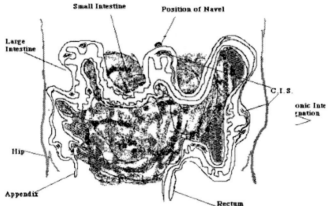

An example of distortion of the arrangement of the Large and Small
Intestines after several years of eating the modern conventional diet.

nall
diet.

Fig. 4

CROSS SECTION OF INTESTINE (General Schematic)
a) Normal.
b) After several years of eating "meat & sugar" diet.

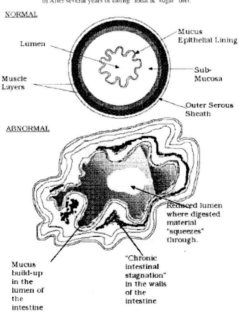

Many different and varied effects arise during the course of this process, chief among them being the gradual loss of the ability of the small intestine to transform chyme into red blood cells. This process is necessarily concomitant with there being a dynamic polarity between the villi and the chyme. However, when the villi are swamped and have been damaged by the mucus buildup, their integrity of function is compromised, and the buildup of mucus has a dampening effect on the polarity of etheric forces between the chyme and the villi, creating insufficient polarity for transformation, which can then no longer take place.

In the case of people in whom chronic intestinal stagnation is gradually occurring, the assimilation of nutrients takes place primarily by diffusion across the semi-permeable membrane of the mucous epithelial lining, through the mucus build-up in the lumen of the intestine, into the bloodstream, and this diffusion occurs less and less efficiently as time goes on.

Then the more yin process of blood formation becomes predominant (since the overall pattern of eating of the present day is overall more yin, we can expect the process of blood formation in most individuals to also be more yin). In modern adults, the bone marrow, skull, ribcage, sternum and spine are the major sites of blood formation; these sites are located in peripheral, upper locations the body, which in terms of position in the body, are more yin sites.

The small intestine and liver are in contrast, more centrally (Δ) located. Furthermore, at the more yin sites, blood formation occurs in a seven-stage process of differentiation (V) of what are called Stem Cells, located throughout the bone marrow (that is, although the above sites predominate more in the more yin formation of red blood cells, any bone marrow can be a site) in which cell division (V) is occurring at every stage, thus producing many red blood cells from one stem cell (a more yin (V) process).

The stages are as follows: the Stem Cell forms the hemocytoblasts, which divide to form basophil erythroblasts, in which production of hemoglobin begins. These become polychromatophil erythroblasts, in which the nucleus of the cells shrinks while still greater amounts of hemoglobin are produced and the cell becomes a normoblast.

Then, when the cytoplasm of the normoblast is filled with hemoglobin to a concentration of 34 percent, the nucleus becomes extremely small and is extruded, forming the reticulocyte. These are so-called because they contain in their cytoplasm remnants of the endoplasmic reticulum, which produces hemoglobin in the earlier stages of cell differentiation; and when the reticulocyte no longer has any reticulum, it is then the red blood cell, or erythrocyte.

In contrast, and as a polarity to the predominately more yang process of assimilation in the person eating daily staple food of cooked whole grains and vegetables, that of transformation of food into blood, in the person eating the fragmented (**V**), refined (**V**), and processed (**V**) modern diet, is a predominantly more yin process of blood formation.

The overall more yin tendency of the modern diet that means the liquid chyme is more yin which, due to the concomitant development of expansion (**V**), fragility (**V**) and turgidity (**V**) of the small intestine which gradually develops as chronic intestine stagnation takes hold over the years of eating the modern diet, means the nutrients in the chyme diffuse (**V**) across the mucus build up and damaged villi into the bloodstream to be carried outward (**V**), upward (**V**), to the peripheral (**V**) bone marrow (**V**), in the hollow (**V**) bone(Δ). Here, many (**V**) stem cells are formed, which differentiate (**V**) and divide (**V**), while becoming smaller (Δ) anucleated (Δ), to form red blood cells (Δ), which make their way into the bloodstream to travel to the center (Δ) the body.

This more yin process of blood formation is the one currently accepted by the scientific community[5]. Whereas the more yang process of transformation of food into blood by the small intestine, is not. This is not surprising, simply because the insight to look into the possibility of transformation of food into blood is denied to the student of hemopoesis, (the scientific term for the study and research of blood formation) due to the fact that research is done on fasting subjects. This necessarily precludes the possibility of food being transformed into blood; since the research subjects at the time studies of are eating no food hemopoesis is being done on them.

According to yin-yang theory, **both** processes of blood formation are occurring in all healthy people, but in the case of people consuming the modern, highly refined (**V**), high fat (**V**), animal protein (**V**), chemically laced (**V**) diet, the more yang process either cannot occur at all, or is reduced to a mere trickle due to the mucus build up the lumen of the small intestine and Chronic Intestinal Stagnation which consequently develops, as already described.

Thus, the blood quality of the modern individual is poor, diffuse, stagnated and fragile. Since the blood is the great mediator of all the organs and tissues of the body—and should be considered an organ itself—as it develops this condition of becoming extremely yin, then the overall dynamics of physiological and metabolic functions of the body are subsequently weakened and enfeebled. The "River of Life" is now thoroughly stagnated and polluted, that is, corrupted, and the consequence symptoms are manifested in all segments and levels of society and in all elements of culture—in its economic condition, social stresses, environmental pollution: in agriculture, commerce, politics, education, medicine etc. Therefore, any realistic attempt toward renewal and healing of earth, culture, and civilization must needs start with the renewal and healing of the quality of blood of the individual as described in this book.

With regard to the same process of chronic intestinal stagnation simultaneously occurring in the large intestine, the consequence is an overall and continuing loss of efficiency of the eliminating functions of the body. I have already detailed how the condition of the large intestine determines the activity and function of the liver, gall bladder, lungs, the kidneys, bladder and skin. Therefore, the development of Chronic Intestinal Stagnation means the subsequent deterioration of functions of all these organs with the consequence of a general and increasing level of the toxicity of the entire organism, manifesting in the process of illness as detailed in previous chapters.

Therefore, it is absolutely critical for individual and the culture, to begin as soon as possible to remove the chronic intestinal stagnation. As this is accomplished a two-fold result will subsequently follow.

One, there will be a re-invigoration of the process of the transformation of food into blood as the dominant means of production of blood, creating a dynamic, vigorous, vital "River of Life"; the refreshed and refreshing blood is transformed into tissue and organ cells, leading to a regeneration, revitalization and healing of the organs and tissues, according to the "wisdom of the body".

And secondly, at the same time, the body's organs of detoxification and elimination will gradually be able to rid the body of the long-standing toxic buildup, which has heretofore occurred.

Although many far-reaching lines of enquiry following through into many domains of human existence may be pursued here, some being hinted at above, these lie outside the scope of this book. All I have endeavored to do thus far, is to show the singular, crucial and all-important role played by the small and large intestines in the onset development and maintenance of all symptomologies of illness, and therefore how these two organs are integrally critical to the healing of the human body, earth and civilization.

NOTES.

1. The ileum and jejunum together constitute the small intestine, there being no appreciable anatomical difference between them.
2. Two points of interest here; one, the surface area the small intestine is equal to the surface area of two football fields; two there are no villi in the large intestine.
3. During the process of transformation of chyme into the red blood cells, one of the most significant substances for the red blood cell, hemoglobin, is a transmutation of chlorophyll, which is found in abundance in leafy greens and other plant foods. Comparing the structure of the two molecules when frozen under a microscope, they are virtually identical, there being some minor differences in the side chains, with the notable exception of the minerals found in the middle or center of each molecule. In the case of chlorophyll it is magnesium, and at the center of hemoglobin is iron; it is theorized here that during the process of transformation of chyme into red blood cells, the magnesium of the chlorophyll molecule is transmuted into the iron of the hemoglobin molecule,
4. In 1979, the East-West Journal, (since renamed Healthy and Natural) published an article by Edward Esko describing the more yang process of blood formation—transformation of food to blood by the small intestine. Some three issues later it published letters from members of the scientific community, whose tone was of angry outrage. I was reading these letters when I received a truly inspiring insight—"Let us quit arguing over who is wrong and who is right. Let us ask the more interesting question—under what circumstances could both theories be correct?"
5. There is a book entitled *Overcoming Cancer* by Dr. Keiichi Morishita (Living Naturally Learning Center, Los Angeles, 1998), which confirms in great detail the process of digestion being the transformation of food into red blood cells.

CHAPTER FIVE

DIAGNOSIS

I stated earlier that in my experience of counseling and teaching over the past 25 years everyone I see, without exception, no matter what their condition or state of health or illness, showed they have Chronic Intestinal Stagnation, and everyone I see on the streets, in coffee bars and restaurants, in newspapers, magazines and on television, in all kinds of activities including professional sports, has Chronic Intestinal Stagnation. It is the universal hallmark of today's culture.

So how can we know the condition of our intestines without having recourse to medical methods of medical diagnosis (and, clearly these are not of much help, because the universal condition of Chronic Intestinal Stagnation in all people of all colors and strata of society has obviously escaped the attention of the medical profession)?

Facial diagnosis.

A beautiful aspect of macrobiotic practice is facial diagnosis. The basics of facial diagnosis can easily be learned by anyone and is without any doubt one of the greatest assets we can acquire for ourselves. In contrast to the highly technological, dehumanized diagnostic techniques of modern medicine, which require highly specialized training, sophisticated and expensive technology, and licensing, facial diagnosis requires study of people faces, something we all do every day, although perhaps without the keenness of attention and attention to detail we need to develop for facial diagnosis. Since facial diagnosis is an art, it is somewhat imprecise. However, its imprecision is more than adequately made up for by its accuracy and timeliness.

Again, to give a description of facial diagnosis in all its details lies outside the scope of this book. I will limit my description to what is "written" in the face which shows we have Chronic Intestinal Stagnation. Figure 1.is a drawing of face which shows the areas of the face which correspond to the large intestine. The primary feature of the face, which shows the condition of the intestines, is the mouth. The upper lip shows the condition of the stomach, the lower lip the condition of the small and large intestines. I described earlier, and the diagram (Chapter 3., Figure3.) shows, the large intestines enclosing or embracing the small intestine.

Fig. 1.

FACIAL DIAGNOSIS FOR INTESTINAL
CONDITION

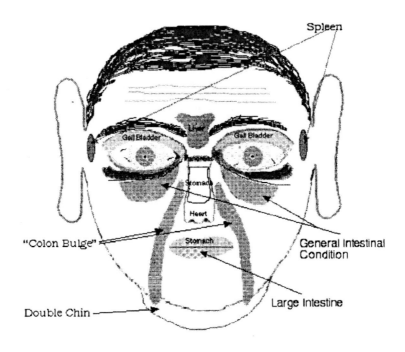

This arrangement holds good in the lower lip, with the outer, visible part of the lip showing the condition of the large intestine; the inner aspect of the lower lip shows the condition of the small intestine. However, I have already described how the process of Chronic Intestinal Stagnation is occurring simultaneously in them both: therefore, if we discern large intestine stagnation we can assume small intestine stagnation is also present.

The essential feature to look for is that the vertical dimension of the upper and lower lip is even in the case of an individual who has healthy, harmonious functioning of the intestinal processes. In Figure 2., A depicts a healthy digestive/eliminative functioning, with the lines X and Y being approximately equal. In B, Y is the longer than X, because the lower lip is swollen relative to the upper lip, revealing Chronic Intestinal Stagnation is present. In this example, the intestinal stagnation is of a more yin nature, that is expanded; if the lower lip is smaller than the upper lip (Y is smaller than X), then the Chronic Intestinal Stagnation is of a more yang (contracted) nature.

Fig. 2.

THE LIPS IN FACIAL DIAGNOSIS.

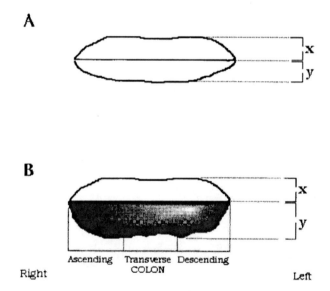

The lower lip can be divided into three equal parts horizontally; the left division corresponds to the ascending (on your face looking into the mirror from your vantage point this will be the right side of the lip) colon[1], the middle division to the transverse, and the right division, the descending colon. There may also be deep vertical lines running down the lower lip, which indicates the presence of diverticulosis.[2] Also there may be discoloration of the skin of the lip—red signifying low grade irritation of large intestine, blue meaning blood stagnation and pale white meaning anemia. Other problems in the large intestine are indicated by the appearance in the skin of the lower lip being chapped and dried, or the presence of various spots, moles, etc.

In the diagram of the face (Figure 1.), the area marked as the Colon Bulge is a swelling running down both sides of the nose, down past the corners of the mouth. A feature common to every human being are lines etched in the skin which run from the corners of the nose and down to the mouth, ending roughly a quarter of an inch from the corner of mouth. If either or, more commonly, both of these lines are deeply etched in the face and is a prominent feature, it is caused by the swelling on the face I term the "colon bulge". This feature, the "colon bulge" indicates Chronic Intestinal Stagnation has become more advanced in the large intestine, (the right side of the face from your point of view looking in the mirror corresponding to the ascending, the left side to the descending colon). This bulge may become so pronounced that sagging of the face occurs and jowls begin to form.

Another indication of intestinal dysfunction is the presence of the feature we call "double chin". The collapse of the flesh under this chin indicates the intestines are relapsing, falling down, that is, collapsing under the weight of the excessive toxic mucus build up in the intestinal walls (Chronic Intestinal Stagnation).

The area marked to the diagram (Figure 1.) under the eye should be distinguished from the area under the eyes, which shows the condition of the kidneys. Every human being has a fine line etched in the skin running from the inner core of the eye, arcing under the eye beneath the lower eyelid to end at a place roughly parallel with the outside corner of the eye. Above this line extending to the lower eyelid is where the condition of the kidneys is seen (left side of the face, left kidney; right side, right kidney). Beneath this line, covering the area marked on the diagram is where the general overall condition of the intestines is seen. Indications of dysfunction in the intestines shown here include swelling, tightness, discoloration of the skin, pimples, spots, moles, nodules, etc.

Another feature of the face every person shows are lines etched horizontally on the forehead. If these lines are prominent, it is because the flesh in the area is swollen, indicating the intestines are swollen.

Additional Diagnostic Features.

Further indications a person has Chronic Intestinal Stagnation are physical, emotional and mental. Anyone experiencing any one or several these features can be positive they have Chronic Intestinal Stagnation. Again, the details of how and why these show that we have Chronic Intestinal Stagnation lie outside the scope of this book, although some of them will hardly need any explanation.

Of course, it is necessary to emphasize and underline here—all illness symptoms of all human beings have their root in the process of Chronic Intestinal Stagnation. The following are those that are directly related to Chronic Intestinal Stagnation.

1. Physical signs.

- Tightness and soreness, hardness in the shoulders, running from the lower area of the neck to the shoulder joints.
- Lower back pain, from where the ribs end to the pelvic bone.
- Lower back spasms and tightness along the lower spine muscles.
- Poor peripheral circulation, causing one's hands and feet to be cold all the time.
- Stiffness, soreness, pain and poor articulation/movement in the lower spine, shoulders and elbows. Tendinitis and ligament pain in these joints.
- Arthritis and bursitis in any joint.
- Frontal headaches and migraine headaches.
- Sciatica
- Pain in the feet, especially the arches, collapsed arches.
- Any type of chronic intestinal discomfort—gas, bloating, diarrhea, constipation, diverticulosis, spastic colon, colitis, malabsorption syndrome, irritable bowel syndrome, Krohn's Disease etc.
- Allergies.
- All sinus conditions.
- Chronic fatigue syndrome, environmental illness, Epstein-Barr virus.
- Parasite infestation of any kind.

Parasites.

A special word on parasitical infections and infestations. These are undoubtedly present in any person with Chronic Intestinal Stagnation; they include worms, bacteria, viruses, amoeba, flagella, spirochetes, funguses, etc. Candidiasis is probably endemic in our society-taking root in the intestinal stagnation in the walls of the intestines, and thus impossible to get rid of unless steps are taken to remove the intestinal stagnation.

It has been estimated the average American carries around in their intestines as much as 4 pounds by weight of toxic parasitical and microbial infestation.

In addition to adopting a macrobiotic dietary practice, and doing the home remedy described later, to get rid of parasites the following anti-parasite remedy is recommended. I must emphasize that this remedy is not done until we have undertaken our macrobiotic dietary practice along with the home remedy program for a minimum of six months

Anti-parasite Remedy.

Dry roast together in a cast iron skillet over medium heat, stirring constantly:
3 cups organic short grain brown rice.
2 cups organic adzuki beans.
1-cup organic brown unhulled sesame seeds.

until the grains of brown rice turn golden brown. Then remove from heat and let cool. Store in a covered glass jar for a minimum of two weeks. If we have poor teeth, we can wait longer after making the remedy, and then when we start chewing, just make sure the mixture is thoroughly mixed with saliva before attempting to chew.

Then for seven days for breakfast, chew one-quarter cup of this mixture as it is, no further cooking is to be done. Do not grind this mixture in a grinder before eating—the necessity for thorough chewing is integral to its effectiveness! After finishing eating, drink a cup of Corsican Seaweed Tea, or make a pot of 1/2 Mugwort: 1/2 Kukicha Twig Tea and drink a cup.

Have your normal macrobiotic lunch and dinner each day while doing the remedy. Repeat this procedure twice more at intervals of two weeks between doing it.

To understand why this remedy is effective is based on yin-yang theory. Relative to the human being, parasites are more yang, and if our condition becomes more yin, our internal environment becomes very attractive to these organisms, which are present everywhere, including our intestines(as referred to above), skin, the air, water, soil, etc. Thus, to rid ourselves of pathogenic organisms, we first have to bring our internal dynamics of physiological/metabolic function back into balance, which takes time.

Then this remedy, being very yang because of the small(Δ), compacted(Δ), dense(Δ) seeds and grains which are dry(Δ) and then roasted(Δ) and then chewed thoroughly(Δ) and then mixed with the most yang substance secreted by the body, our saliva. From yin-yang theory we know yang repels yang, so when we ingest this mixture after thorough chewing, pathogenic organisms of every hue and form in the body are either destroyed or they leave the body forthwith[4].

- Insomnia.
- Any skin condition, including dandruff, psoriasis, eczema, impetigo, etc.
- Loss of hair on the top front part of the head.
- Bad breath and body odor, flatulence
- In women all female organ conditions of any description, in the ovaries, fallopian tubes, uterus, vagina, and breasts, have their origin in Chronic Intestinal Stagnation is my observation when working with women

over the past 25 years. This is because simultaneously with the Chronic Intestinal Stagnation going on in the intestines, a similar process is taking place in the uterine walls.
- In women, any thyroid condition.

2. Emotional signs.

The emotional signature of Chronic Intestinal Stagnation is depression, and in extreme cases, manic depression.

- Anorexia and Bulimia.
- Chronic melancholy and sadness. Strictly speaking these have more to do with the lungs, but since the lungs are the paired organs of the large intestines, the intestinal stagnation is accompanied by lung stagnation.

3. Mental signs.

- Thinking tends to be foggy, scattered and unclear, and one cannot mentally concentrate for any great length of time.
- Attention deficit disorder.
- Manic depression or depression.
- The tendency toward procrastination.
- The difficulty of putting into action any project or idea one has; if one does start something, difficulty in seeing it through to its completion.
- Difficulty in arising out of bed in the morning.
- Poor function of the will activity. This means a person has difficulty, and is resistant to, doing anything that requires a significant change in their usual, daily normal life patterns. By life patterns, I mean habitual modes of thinking, feeling and doing.

NOTES

1. Colon is another word for the large intestine.
2. Diverticulosis a condition of the intestines where the intestinal walls have weakened to the point deep pockets form in the wall, where old fecal matter and stagnated mucus, and other detritus gather over the years. It is a precursor of colon cancer. In the US, one out of every five people over the age of 40 has diverticulosis, three out of every five people over the age of 70.
3. Of course the state of bowel movement is the eloquent signifier of the condition of the intestines. I will spare the reader descriptions of the wide variations of intestinal disharmony reflected in bowel movement. Suffice it to say, on a generally consistent basis, intestinal digestive harmony is reflected in the colon emptying itself once daily in approximately 30-45 seconds, between 7.00-9.00 a.m. The stools are a light brown color, have a slight aromatic smell, are well formed with consistent texture and float in the water of the toilet
4. In a healthy human organism, the intestinal microflora are very significant in many ways, including repairing the intestinal wall, secreting enzymes important in digestion and in producing B vitamins and assisting in the assimilation of these B vitamins into the blood.

CHAPTER SIX

THE GINGER COMPRESS

If we have established beyond reasonable doubt that we do have Chronic Intestinal Stagnation, then we may want to inquire as to what we can do to aid our intestines in healing themselves. From what has already been written it should be fairly clear we must first needs begin by changing our way of eating to one based on eating cooked whole grains and vegetables[1]. However, on the physical level, changing our way of eating is not enough. It is often assumed, at least it appears to be the assumption, in macrobiotic literature, we need but change our daily staple foods from meat, eggs, dairy food, refined, chemicalized foods, etc. to cooked whole grains and vegetables and our intestinal function will take care of itself. And, in many instances, when people begin eating whole grain and vegetables according to macrobiotic principles, one of the first changes noticed is a considerable, often dramatic improvement in bowel movement.

However, the consumption of these foods—cooked whole grains and vegetables—on a regular basis as staple foods does not allow for making any real inroads on breaking down the Chronic Intestinal Stagnation, the toxic mucus build-up in the intestinal walls. The Chronic Intestinal Stagnation has, as has already been suggested, been going on over the entire life of the individual living in modern culture, eating the modern diet, and as the years go by the Chronic Intestinal Stagnation becomes extraordinarily impacted and "locked-in" the intestinal walls. Thus we must do something in addition to changing our way of eating if we wish to get rid of the toxic mucus stagnation in the walls of our intestines.

I must avow I am not the first person in the history of humanity to recognize the large intestines as the single most critical organ to address if we wish to affect a true and deep healing of the body. Many, many treatments have been devised over the years in an attempt to remove this impacted mucus material, including enemas, colonics, clay treatments, herbal colon cleansing programs, and fasts of innumerable kinds and varieties. However, none of them actually work in removing the Chronic Intestinal Stagnation, which is lodged in the walls of the intestines. Many are difficult to do, and some actually detrimental. For example, I think, colonics actually weaken the walls of the intestines.

These treatments are effective in sloughing off the mucus build-up in the lumen or cavity of the intestines, but then so is eating a diet based on cooked whole grains and vegetables due to the high fiber content of these foods.

The most effective remedy of which I know is probably several thousand years old, and was probably devised at the beginning of recorded history. I have also heard it was thought up by a physician of a Buddhist persuasion around 500 BC. No matter. To the august and profoundly wise gentleman or gentlewoman who first came up with the idea of the ginger compress, I offer my profound prayer of gratitude.

So, after a long and necessary preliminary discourse, we come to the reason for the writing of this book:

The Ginger Compress.

Items required:

1. One gallon of water in a container with a lid (tap water is fine).
2. One quarter of cup finely grated—**by hand**—fresh, unpeeled ginger root (non-organic is fine) wrapped in the cheesecloth, or other natural fiber cloth, to make a bag of grated ginger[2]. A ginger root, which fits in the palm of your hand, will suffice for the amount of grated ginger needed.
3. Two one foot wide terry cloth towels three feet long. Also good are cotton baby diapers.
4. One cotton bath towel,
5. One pair of thick rubber gloves.

Preliminaries.

Before proceeding, take the terry cloth towels and, singly, fold each one in three-fold such that it covers the area of your abdomen, which goes from the sternum (breastbone) of the rib cage to the pelvic bone, and from one hip to the other hip. Once you've done this, sew each one along the loose edges so they are prevented from falling open once you start doing the treatment.

Also, the treatment has to be done on an empty stomach, either an hour before you eat or two hours after you eat. It can be done at any time of day. However, a practical tip is to do the treatment before you go to bed, and after doing it, leave all the materials where they are in the kitchen, and go to bed. First thing in the morning, before eating breakfast, reheat the ginger water pot, making sure you do not boil the water, and you can do the treatment again. Thus you can use one pot of ginger water for two treatments.

If we use one gallon container for our ginger compress then after it is ready to start doing the treatment, the ginger water will retain its heat long enough to do two, possibly three, treatments before needing to be reheated. If you want to ensure the ginger water remains hot after you have taken it off the stove, obtain a hot plate you can plug into an electrical outlet near the place you choose to do the treatment and place the pot of ginger water on it after you have made it.

Instructions.

METHOD ONE.

Place the container of water on the stove and bring the water to a boil. Meanwhile, grate the unpeeled ginger root using a fine tooth grater (do **not** use a blender) until you have approximately one quarter cup of grated ginger; the easiest way to assure you do not lose any ginger root is to place the piece of cloth you're using to wrap the ginger in, in a bowl and grate the ginger onto the cloth in the bowl.

When you have grated enough ginger, bring the four corners of the cloth in the bowl together to enclosed the grated ginger in the cloth; twirl to make a neck and wrap a rubber band or tie around the neck to hold the four corners together. You now have a bag of ginger. Any ginger juice will be found at the bottom of the bowl.

By now the water in the pot will be near to boiling, if it has not already reached boiling. Then, and this is the most important point, once the water has reached boiling point, switch your heat source off and let the water stop boiling **before** taking the bag of grated ginger, squeezing the excess juice in the grated ginger into the hot water, place the bag in the pot, and if there is any ginger juice in the bowl you grated the ginger into, pour that in also.

Then place the two folded and sewn up terry cloth towels or cotton diapers in the pot of hot ginger water and let them soak for a minute or two, with the lid of the container on.

You are now ready to do the compress.

Place an old blanket or sheet on your couch, carpet or bed, wherever you choose to do the compress and set up the pot of ginger water with the two terry cloth towels (henceforth referred to as the ginger towels) in it, on some newspapers within easy reach of where you lie down on your back (do not use plastic in any shape or form) on the couch, bed or floor, expose the skin of your abdomen, and place the bath towel, also folded so it can cover your abdomen, on your lap.

Then, with the rubber gloves on your hands, remove the lid of the pot, place it on the floor, and take up one of the ginger towels in the pot (if you're lying on the floor you need to sit up to do this), ring out the excess liquid into the pot, then replace the lid on the pot to keep the heat in.

Taking the wrung-out ginger towel, open it up so it is flat (it will remain folded if you have sewn the loose edges together), lie down if you had to sit up to do the preceding, and raise and lower the ginger towel over the skin of your abdomen, close to but not actually touching the skin to begin with[3], until you can tolerate the ginger towel laid directly on the skin. After you have placed the hot ginger towel directly on the skin of your abdomen, cover it with the bath towel, which has been lying on your lap, to keep the heat in.

After two to five minutes the ginger towel on your abdomen will start to cool down. Then, lift up the bath towel covering the ginger towel; remove the cooled ginger towel, leaving the bath towel so it covers the abdomen to keep it warm.

Remove the lid from the ginger water pot, place the just used wet, cooled ginger towel back in it to reheat it, and remove the second ginger towel, which has been soaking in the ginger pot while you were using the first ginger towel. Thoroughly ring out the excess ginger water in this second towel back into the container, replace the lid and repeat the procedure as with the first ginger towel. Alternate the two ginger towels in this manner for half an hour. This constitutes one treatment.

Treatment instructions.

I recommend the compress be done 64 times, two to four times a week. This constitutes one round of compresses; this may not be, and is generally not, enough to complete the rehabilitation of our intestines[4].

If you determine your intestines need more work, I suggest waiting for 6-8 weeks and then do another round of 64 compresses. I think it takes three rounds of 64 compresses each, generally speaking, to complete the rehabilitation of our intestines. I also recommend that the three rounds of 64 compresses each be done over a one to two-year period.

It must not to be assumed that doing more ginger compresses more often is better than I recommend here. The intestines undergo their rehabilitation in their own good time, so we must show patience in allowing them to do so. In my experience it takes a minimum of two years for the intestines to rehabilitate themselves and a maximum of seven years. It is also important to point out that the 64 compresses per round doing to 2-4 compresses a week is not mandatory. What I mean is it is important to do the 64 compresses per round. However, it is not always possible to do compresses every week because you may be on vacation, or for work or some other reason you do not have the time in a particular week or two. Therefore it is fine to miss doing it for one or two weeks; just taking up where you left off, keeping track of the amount of compresses you have already done.

The reason it takes so many compresses to complete the rehabilitation of our intestines is the Chronic Intestinal Stagnation has developed over many, many years, even decades. The older we are when we discover our Chronic Intestinal Stagnation, the longer it has been going on. And the longer it has been going on, the more tenaciously hardened and impacted it is in our intestinal walls. Therefore the more ginger compresses we'll have to do, more consistently and with perseverance, in order for the compresses to have their desired effects.

I also recommend that once you are satisfied your intestines are back in shape again, it is a good idea to do ten to twenty compresses every few years, although this will depend upon you doing your facial diagnosis to determine the condition of your intestines. With regard to children it is better to wait until they are seven years old before doing the ginger compress regimen on them[5].

METHOD TWO.

This method I learned from David Jackson, a macrobiotic teacher and counselor living in Arizona.—the following description is his:

1. Large stockpot with lid 3/4 full of boiling water just removed from the stove.
2. 1/4 cup of raw grated ginger (A) (unpeeled) in cotton cloth or washcloth—tied (B)
3. 2-cotton diapers, 1 cotton towel, 1 wooden spoon or chopstick
4. 2 wooden bowls 8-10 inches in diameter that fit inside each other closely

Grating the ginger root onto a cotton muslin cloth:

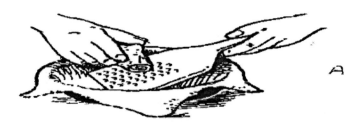

The ready to use bag of Grated Ginger Root.

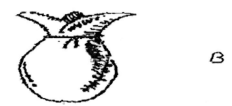

Squeeze the ginger bag (B) between the 2 bowls (C) so that the juice goes into the hot water pot (1).

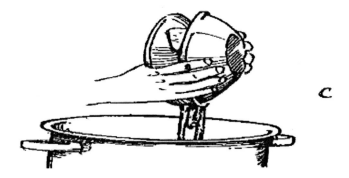

Dip the ginger bag into the water several times and squeeze again. Finally, drop the ginger bag into the water and leave it there to continue to strengthen the liquid. Always cover the pot when not dipping into it to maintain the heat. This pot now is your ginger pot.

Find a comfortable spot on the floor against a wall or such with a couple of big pillows behind you to rest against. Place the hot ginger pot alongside you on a thick cloth or rug to keep the heat from being dispersed. Lie on your back and expose your tummy fully.

Fold 1 dry diaper (3) in half and place it over the abdominal area (from the top of the pubic bone to the sternum. Place the second diaper in the ginger pot. Place the towel folded on the thighs. Dip into the ginger pot with the wooden utensil (3) and fetch the diaper. Place the wet diaper between the 2 bowls and squeeze the excess liquid back into the pot (C) and cover the pot to keep it hot. Place the hot wet squeezed diaper (folded in half) on top of the dry one (which is on the abdomen) and cover both with the towel to keep the warmth in. If the diapers become too hot against the body, lift them slightly until the body becomes used to it. As the body feels comfortable, flip the diapers so that the hotter one is now against the skin. Finally, take the (now cooler) top diaper and place it into the ginger pot to refresh it for a minute or so. Remove it again from the pot and squeeze it between the 2 bowls again to remove excess liquid and place it on top of the remaining diaper on the abdomen (keep the top on the pot). As soon as the body can handle the heat, flip the diapers so the hotter one is against the body again. Continue with this keeping the body as hot as you can handle it for about 30 minutes. Continue to keep the towel covering the diapers on the body to keep the heat in between diaper activity. The abdomen usually becomes reddish with the increased blood circulation—that's great!

The activity of ginger is amazing. It is a root (downward energy), which also has a very strong dispersing odor when grated (upward energy). This dynamic quality enhances heat and activity. The strong downward presence during the compress penetrates deep into the organs as well as through the walls of the organs. The dispersing effect increases circulation ten fold and assists in breaking up hardened accumulation which could be 50 years old or more. The increased circulation also assists in eliminating these excesses from the body and returning the body's natural rhythms to normal. Eating well during this time is important, as you do not want to slow down this process. Also discharges may occur during this process and you may want to consult your counselor during these times. Do not use on the brain, on infants, during high fevers or pregnancy, or on any direct inflammation or cancerous area.

The Activity of the Ginger Compress.

The ginger compress works because of the etheric or chi activities of the heat and the ginger root. From the perspective of yin-yang theory, the ginger root has strong yang activity by virtue its "rootness". This more yang activity means the etheric activity of the ginger has a strong, downward, penetrating direction of movement.

On the other hand when we grate the ginger root we notice how the aroma of ginger powerfully fills the room, attesting to the strong dispersing, expansive movement of ginger chi. The reason for this is the ginger root grows horizontally under the ground, which means it is also influenced by more yin activity, than, for example, burdock or carrot roots which grow straight down. It this additional more yin factor that is responsible for its dispersing (more yin) activity, which is further enhanced by finely grating the ginger.

My feeling is that by doing the ginger compress in this way, laying the towel soaked in the hot ginger water, which is permeated with the etheric activity of the ginger root, thereby harnessing it, on the abdomen while lying on our back, the ginger towel focuses these etheric forces on the abdominal cavity, in which the intestines lie, and they penetrate into the tissues by means of the root (more yang) activity and break up the toxic mucus stagnation encountered in the tissues by means of the strong dispersive activity. Furthermore, the etheric forces of the ginger stimulate the etheric forces of the intestines, thus activating their proper activity[6].

The activity of the heat of the compress stimulates the circulation of the blood and tissue fluids in the area being treated, which then facilitates the bearing of the dispersed toxins away to be excreted.

The combination of these three etheric or "chi" activities brought to bear by the compress, means the tissues of the walls of the intestines begin to receive clean, revitalized blood (if we have also changed our way of eating to a daily fare of cooked whole grains and vegetables, and it has to be emphasized the ginger compresses are wasted time if we have not) for the first time in years, or decades. They become revitalized, leading to a regeneration of the tissues and restoration of their proper, harmonious function.

During The Treatments.

As a result of doing the treatments, toxic mucus deposits are gradually dissolved and flushed into the bloodstream, and what happens overtly as a consequence will depend on many factors.

All I will say here, and more will be said on this subject in the chapter "Macrobiotic Healing", is that the body may show signs of detoxification or may show no overt signs of it cleansing itself other than passive weight loss, increased urination and bowel movement and some fatigue.

More active signs of cleansing include nasal mucus discharges, sore throat, coughing and sneezing, fever, and flu-like symptoms, temporary constipation and/or diarrhea, various aches and pains, skin eruptions in various parts of body and headaches. If accompanied with healthy appetite, normal sleep patterns, general vitality and no nausea, these signs indicate the healing process is going very well.

Contra-indications.

The ginger compress on the abdomen should not be done in the following instances:

> During pregnancy and breast-feeding. It can be done when menstruating.
> If there is abdominal inflammation, peritonitis, pneumonia.
> On the brain.
> On infant babies.
> In cases where a high fever is running.
> If there is presence of overt cancers in the abdominal region, although they may safely be done if cancer is present in other parts of the body.

In macrobiotic literature, which discuss the ginger compress, you will come across writings on "*special considerations for cancer patients . . .*" and there is mention of the Taro Potato Plaster. The reason it is mentioned that cancer patients should not do the ginger compress for more than five minutes on the cancer is because it is thought the stimulation of the blood supply caused by the compress means that, if there is a cancerous tumor in the region being treated, the increased blood circulation will cause the cancer to grow.

However, this is only true if the blood is still toxic. When a person starts a macrobiotic dietary regimen, in ten days the blood plasma (the fluid in which the blood circulates) is renewed; in 30-60 days all the white blood cells will be newly created, and in 120 days all the red blood cells will be newly created.

Thus, theoretically, if we begin the ginger compresses four months after starting the dietary practice, then the increasing blood flow means clean, revitalized, fresh blood will be circulating more vigorously. The cancer consequently will then be receiving this fresh clean blood, which in turn means the cancer will dissolve faster. However, to act on the side of caution, if a person has cancer of the colon or some other cancer of the abdominal region, it is perhaps wiser to wait until the macrobiotic practice has been done for one year before embarking on the regimen of ginger compresses.

I have also heard comments the regimen of two to four compresses a week applies too much heat to the organs being treated. However, doing it the maximum four times to the abdominal region is a total of two hours of the 168 hours of the week, which comes to 1.19 percent of the week, hardly excessive.

Furthermore if we classify all illnesses of the human organism into two groups; whether they are illnesses from too much heat, or illnesses from too much cold, in the body, then it turns out of all the degenerative illnesses are illnesses of too much cold in the body.

Two problems may become evident during the course of the treatments. One is that the skin of the abdomen takes on a darkened, brown-red /yellow hue; this will clear up after regimen has been completed. The other is the possibility of detoxifying too rapidly; meaning the symptoms of discharge may become overwhelming. In this case, simply adjust the rhythm of the compresses by temporarily stopping them for a few days or a week or two. The key point, as I pointed out before, about the regimen of 64 compresses is to do them; whether this takes 16, 20, 32 or 40 weeks is immaterial; what is required is to get the compresses done on a relatively consistent basis and to complete the 64.

The Daikon Hip Bath.

In the case of women, do the ginger compress on the abdomen twice a week. As I have already mentioned previously it is my observation that women who have Chronic Intestinal Stagnation also have, concurrently, chronic uterine wall stagnation. Doing an additional home remedy, the daikon hipbath, immeasurably helps this female organ condition.

The daikon hipbath is referred to in macrobiotic literature as the universal remedy for all female organ conditions and I recommend it be done twice a week along with two times a week of ginger compresses. This means a total of 32 daikon hip baths and a total of 32 ginger compresses are done over a period of 16-20 weeks or more as the case may be. These remedies are absolutely to no avail if they are not also accompanied by changing to a macrobiotic dietary practice.

Items needed.

> A one-gallon container with a lid filled with 1/2-gallon water.
> The dried leaves of 4 bunches daikon greens.
> One handful of sea salt

If you cannot obtain daikon greens, then use either turnip leaves or comfrey leaves. In all cases the greens must be hung to dry in a place away from direct sunlight until the leaves become crisp and dry before using them. It is possible the grocery store from which you obtain your vegetables sells the daikon radish. If they do, ask the grocery manager of the store to save a bag of the greens for you (usually the greens are cut off before the daikon radishes are put on display). Take them home and dry them by hanging them up on a piece of string in your garage or attic or other suitable place in the shade.

Instructions.

The treatment has to be done at night before going to bed. Once you get in the bath to do the treatment you must go to bed immediately after getting out of the bath.

Place the container with the water along with the four bunches of dried daikon leaves in the water, bring to boil and let simmer for half an hour. Add a generous handful of sea salt or rock salt.

Then run a hot bath, so that you can lie in it with the water up to your neck, or you can sit in the bath with the water up to your navel, and the upper part of your body wrapped with a towel to keep it warm. Then pour the salty daikon water into the bath through a strainer or sieve to keep the leaves out of the bath. These are later discarded.

Get in the bath, with the water as comfortably hot as you can stand it, and soak for fifteen to twenty minutes. Then get out, and dry yourself off rapidly, get well covered by, as a suggestion, wearing pajamas, a dressing gown and a scarf on your head and socks on your feet and go to bed.

Activity of the dried daikon leaves.

The activity of the dried daikon leaves, because of the upward movement of the leaves as they are growing, and shrinking activity as they are dried, means these dynamics are in the water when you get into the bath.

The result is the etheric or "chi" activity of the daikon leaves prepared in this manner cuts through the fatty, mucus deposits in the uterine walls, ovaries, fallopian tubes and breasts (even if you're not lying the bathtub up to your neck) and dissolves them, drawing the dissolved fatty mucus along with the toxins down toward the uterus to be excreted in the form, usually, of vaginal discharge. The heat of the bath stimulates the overall blood and tissue fluid circulation so that after you get into bed, you will eventually begin to sweat, sometimes profusely.

Of course, some women may begin to sweat on the first occasion of doing the bath, but more usually it takes several weeks because most women have a lot of fat accumulated in the skin and this needs to be dissolved first before real sweating can begin.

The results from doing the daikon bath brings about, if, and only if accompanied by change to a macrobiotic dietary regimen of cooked whole grains and vegetables, the following:

A cleansing and tonification of all the female organs.

A thoroughgoing cleansing of the skin, including facial skin, which is truly remarkable to see.

The dissolving and melting way of fat deposits everywhere in the body.

Therefore, it is used in all conditions of the breasts, ovaries, fallopian tubes and the uterus/vagina, for helping to lose weight, and as a tremendous skin cleaner, as long as we have also changed our eating habits to a macrobiotic way of eating.

Cautionary Remarks.

This home remedy is only to be done by women. Again, for girls, please wait until they are 7 years old before doing them.

Do not do the Daikon Bath if there is presence of any heart condition requiring medication; in this case, from a macrobiotic perspective, get on a macrobiotic way of eating for four to six months, then gradually wean yourself off the medication over a period of 6-8 weeks, with the guidance of an experienced macrobiotic counselor, and then start the Daikon Bath home remedy. (In my experience it is remarkable how quickly the heart heals itself with a macrobiotic way of eating).

Also, if one is breast-feeding, it is advised to do the daikon bath after the baby has been weaned.

It is a good idea, say for the first three to four weeks of doing the bath, to not schedule anything for the day after doing the bath. In the beginning weeks of doing the bath you tend to feel somewhat fatigued to being very tired the day after doing it and is better to relax and take it easy. Also, if it happens that the cleansing of the female organs manifests as vaginal discharge and/or symptoms similar to those which manifest in urinary tract infections such as burning and itching and urinating frequently, then the following macrobiotic home remedy will help to alleviate discomfort.

Umeboshi Plum Douche.

Place the flesh of 6-7 umeboshi plums in one quart of water and bring to a boil. Switch the heat off and let cool to body temperature. Then strain out one cup of the umeboshi liquid and use to douche. The next day, reheat the water to reach body temperature and douche again with one cup of the umeboshi liquid. Repeat daily until the liquid is gone; add three to four more umeboshi plums to the ones already in the pot, and another quart of water. Bring to a boil and repeat the procedure. Do this for ten days, douching once a day.

Black Soybean Tea.

This is another helpful home remedy specifically for the female organs:

Dry roast one-quarter cup black soybeans in a saucepan stirring
constantly for five minutes.

Add two cups of water.

Bring to a boil and let simmer, with the lid off, until half the water has
evaporated and one cup of liquid is left in the saucepan. Strain
out the beans. (eat them after they having undergone further
cooking, perhaps another 30 minutes, adding a pinch of sea salt
at the end of cooking so they can be digested properly).

Add 1/4 teaspoonful of tamari or soy sauce to the one cup black
soybean tea.

Drink a 1/3 cup a day for three days, reheating each time (store in
refrigerator).

Repeat once a week, three days each week, for a total of six weeks.

Possible hindrances to doing the ginger compress.

I've noticed, over the course of counseling thousands of individuals, that there is
a great deal of resistance to actually doing the ginger compresses. I estimate perhaps
30 percent of the people I counsel actually do the two to three rounds of compresses
necessary to completely dissolve and breakup the Chronic Intestinal Stagnation.

Of course, people say they do not have the time; it's too complicated, or some
other excuse. The true reasons are, I feel, a lot deeper. First, the intestines are those
organs of the body that have to do with the expression of the activities of the will forces
of the soul; will forces have to do with carrying out actions and completing them.

If the intestines are weak and stagnated, then when we are asked to do
something, which requires a significant and radical change in any one of our
habitual ways of doing any activity or in our day-to-day life routine, we find
this very difficult to do. The ginger accomplish regimen requires we take into
account our necessity for doing them.

This means we need to schedule the times, consciously, to do them during
the course of the week. If we do not do this, then we will have difficulty in
getting them started, let alone completed.

Secondly, the large intestines and the lungs correspond to the forebrain; and
the forebrain is the sense—organ for the thinking activity of the soul. Thus, if
we have Chronic Intestinal Stagnation, we also have toxic mucus buildup in
the lungs and our forebrain is also stagnated.

In regard to thinking, this means our thinking is stuck, molded in the tried
and old, habitual, received learning we have picked from the school, college, the
church, from our family and through the newspapers and mass media.

If we are to break through the arid, stagnated, arid, destructive techno—
material thinking of modern culture, we have to break up the stagnation in the
forebrain while at the same time undertaking the strenuous re-education and
quest for self knowledge necessary for true healing to occur. The ginger compress

regimen on the intestines is fundamentally necessary if we are to achieve this, and this is an uncomfortable prospect, at least, sub-consciously.

Thirdly, and, probably the most difficult of the three impediments to overcome, is our emotional makeup. In the course of counseling I have come across a remarkable phenomenon of human life.

The phenomenon I have observed is that when we experience a deeply wounding event during the course of childhood or young adult life, like being sexually abused, or physically or mentally/emotionally beaten down, the events which occasion these traumas and abuses are actually recorded or "imprinted" in the mucus stagnation, in any organ or tissue the body where the mucus stagnation happens to develop.

That is to say, the mucus stagnation acts as a medium in which the events in question are holographically imprinted. This means that no matter how well we succeed in suppressing our memory of these events, they are literally playing out continuously, like an endless tape loop, for as long as the mucus stagnation remains in the body.

Thus, there is not only the detrimental physical consequence of increasing toxicity of the body resulting from the mucus build-up of Chronic Intestinal Stagnation, which, as I have shown, starts with a large and small intestines (and, because these organs relationship are complimentary with the lungs and heart, occurs in those organs too), there are also emotional consequences.

It is helpful at this juncture to look at the Five Transformation Theory, which describes the relationships of the more destructive emotions with the organs in a toxic condition as follows:

Liver/Gall Bladder—frustration, irritability, impatience and anger.
Kidney/Bladder—fear, anxiety, loss of confidence and self-esteem.
Lungs—melancholy and sadness, a sense of loss.
Large intestine—depression, loss of enthusiasm, boredom.
Heart/Small Intestine—over excitability, nervousness, hysteria.
Stomach/Spleen—Pancreas—doubt, worry, skepticism, cynicism.

These emotional moods are, in the person so afflicted, permanent and cannot be explained by any current events in their lives. They are, so to speak, their mood of soul, and color every motivation, attitude, expression and way of relating to themselves and the people in their lives and the world in which they live.

They are permanent, that is, for as long as the mucus stagnation is present, in which emotional trauma are imprinted. I must point out of these "permanent moods of soul" are present as long as the physical stagnation is present, even if there have not been any emotional traumas in a person's life

However, it is probable that if there have been emotional traumas—and it is fairly evident that emotional, mental, physical and sexual abuse is widely prevalent in modern culture—the imprinting of the events occasioning these traumas has the effect of accentuating their mood of soul to a deeper extent than in those individuals who have been fortunate enough not to have been emotionally, physically or sexually abused in early childhood and early adulthood.

When we do the ginger compresses on our abdomen, then the dissolution of mucus stagnations will cause the "holographically imprinted event" to be released from its entrapment in the mucus stagnations, as the latter is dissolved by the ginger compresses, these events will surface into our consciousness and we'll have to deal with them psychologically and emotionally.

It is probable, and I have observed this in several people with whom I've been working, that when these events surface into our consciousness, it is the first time they became aware that these events had even occurred, as they had done such an effective job of suppressing their memory of these events when they did occur.

This dawning of consciousness and remembering of the traumatic event(s) is, in many instances, a traumatic experience, as can well be understood, occasioning much pain and suffering. I feel when people are suggested to do the ginger compresses, they know, subconsciously, the dissolving of the mucus stagnations (thereby releasing the "holographically imprinted event") as a result of doing the compresses, and since the pain and trauma associated with these events are so profound, people would rather not have to deal with them. Thus, they have a subconscious resistance to doing the ginger compress regimen.

This is understandable. However, any healing that is worthy of the name is necessarily going to be accompanied with pain and suffering; this is unavoidable. If we go through a healing that leads to a resolution of our symptoms, but which is not accompanied with pain and suffering, whether physical, emotional or mental, then we can be assured the healing is superficial and will not bring about the profound transformation of our being, in body, soul and spirit which is the healing I am discussing in this writing.

The ginger compresses then, though are often psychologically, to a great degree, and to some degree physically, painful, they need to be done if we wish to bring about a true and deep healing of ourselves and the world in which we live.

As to what I feel we need to do if we realize we have been physically, emotionally, mental or sexually abused in childhood and early adulthood, I offer the following suggestions:

1. No blame. I do not feel that blaming the perpetrators of these traumas helps anyone; no matter how justified we may feel in so doing.

Furthermore, any idea of vengeance and revenge simply does not answer the questions posed by these events and leaves out of account the most important fact of human spiritual life. This is karma. Karma is a profound spiritual reality that is not taking into account at all in their day-to-day lives by people living today. Now, karma is a vast subject, and all I will say here is karma means that inexorably, ineluctably, without regard to our station in life, we have to make up to others, either in this lifetime, or some subsequent life on earth, in one way or another what we have done to them. This is called atonement. Thus, it is not our position to make personal judgments (if it is a question of the law, that is another matter), for everyone's misdeeds will be accounted for through their personal karma[7].

2. Forgiveness. We must dig deep in our souls and find it possible to forgive the individual(s) involved for what has been done, not as a cursory nod to the idea of forgiving, but as a profound reality in our souls.

3. Find something about the event or the individuals involved which is beautiful and good; for it is rare for any one individual or event to be irredeemably evil.

    This is probably the most difficult suggestion to carry through, and also the most important; to ask ourselves what was it about ourselves that occasioned these events to take place. What is it that we need to work on,—mentally, emotionally, spiritually—so we can truly digest and learn the lessons needing to be learnt from these events for ourselves.

4. Once we have digested and learned all that needs to be learnt and understood and are making the changes in ourselves, forget about the events, release them, for time itself is a great healer. As healthy human beings, we cannot remain trapped in the past or live vicariously in the future, only in the present.

Additional Aids.

Here are some additional ways to aid breaking up the chronic mucus stagnation in our intestines. The first is to make sure we go for a walk at least half to one hour 5-6 days a week. The act of walking serves as an internal massage on the intestines. It is helpful to use the stairs instead of the elevator or escalator; to walk to the store rather than to drive etc. Walking is most helpful if it is a relaxed stroll around the neighborhood or at the park, where the aim is simple enjoyment of the sights and sounds we encounter on our walk, rather than trying to do any intense exercise.

Also helpful is massaging the intestines while doing the compress. While lying on our back with the ginger towel on our abdomen, using our extended index and middle finger of both hands together, press on the intestines beginning at the ileo-cecal valve approximately 2 inches to the left of the right hip bone,.

Using a push and release motion, work your fingers up the right side of the abdomen, across the abdomen to the left, just above the navel, and then down the left side of the abdomen to just above the pelvic bone. Then, moving inward in a spiraling motion, further in from the path you have just traversed, work in toward the center of the abdomen. When you have completed one massage in this way, start again from beginning and work your fingers to the center again. Do this two to three times or more during the time you're doing the compress. When you press down your fingers, go as deep as you can, while trying to keep the abdominal muscles completely relaxed.

Another aid is the following exercise. Stand up straight, eyes looking straight ahead, with your hands by your side, in the middle of a room so you have plenty of space to move. Then move your hands, fingers extended, upward and outward while raising yourself up on your toes while taking a deep breath through your nose so the in-breath goes into your lower abdomen.

Hold this the position momentarily, then slowly, simultaneously, bring both hands down past the hips and then forward in front of you while bending down into a "skiing" position, tightening your abdominal and buttock muscles as you bend. Exhale slowly through your mouth, in order to complete the exhalation of all the air in your lungs as you end up in the "skiing" position. What I mean by the skiing position is you end up the exercise on your toes, bent at the waist with the buttocks close to the ankles, arms extended in front you with the fingers extended forward, as if you were just about to push off down a slope if you were wearing skis.

What you will feel if you do this motion properly is a gathering and a concentration of chi or etheric forces in the pit of the abdomen, Do this exercise, on an empty stomach, three to five times each session, two to four times a week while you are doing the ginger compress regimen.

Tai Chi and Yoga are also beneficial. Any form of strenuous exercise is not recommended during the first year of changing over to a macrobiotic way of eating. The reason is, during the early stages of being on a macrobiotic regimen, the body is detoxifying itself and the organs of detoxification and elimination are actively carrying out the dissolving and removal of mucus and toxins.

When we do any form of strenuous exercise, like jogging, high-impact aerobics, weight-lifting etc., then our metabolic rate increases, meaning more toxins of cellular activity are being generated than when our metabolism is functioning normally. Therefore, the organs of detoxification and elimination of wastes are being asked to deal with the detoxification and elimination of wastes, which occurs as a result of starting a macrobiotic dietary regimen, as well as with the additional toxins created by intense physical exercise.

This does put a heavy strain on these organs which are at best in a weakened and fragile condition when we start our macrobiotic dietary program and the added load caused by the heavy exercise makes it a lot more difficult for these organs, in doing both jobs of detoxification and elimination, and at the same time, regenerating and revitalizing themselves. Therefore strenuous exercise is avoided for at least a year.

NOTES.

1. This subject is addressed in more detail in the chapter on General Dietary Recommendations.
2. The reason for placing the grated ginger in a bag is to avoid having pieces of ginger floating about in the water or getting on the towels. Also, if ginger is boiled, the treatments will not work.
3. If you place the ginger towel immediately on the skin you will scald the skin, a very painful experience!
4. You can check the facial features described in the chapter on diagnosis to see what changes occur. To make this easy, I recommend you have a photograph taken of your face before starting the regimen of ginger compresses, and another one after you've completed the 64 treatments. If you do this, you will get a much clearer impression of the changes by comparing the "before" and "after" photographs side by side.
5. Children today are being born with Chronic Intestinal Stagnation, due to the "modern diets" of their mothers during pregnancy.
6. When we cover the abdomen from the sternum to the pubic bone, we are also treating the stomach and spleen/ pancreas, and the liver/gallbladder, and because the lungs are the paired complimentary organs of the large intestine, and heart of the small intestine, these organs are also being treated.
7. Rudolf Steiner has given many lectures on karma, and I urge the reader get hold of Volumes 1-8 of his series of lectures entitled Karmic Relationships (Rudolf Steiner Press, London).

CHAPTER SEVEN

INTERLUDE

At this juncture of the book it will be helpful to take a pause and look over what has been written, to amplify and emphasize the essential points that have been made.

Rudolf Steiner made the remark in one of his lectures on August 11th, 1919, that "we needed radically different heads on our shoulders."[1]. This is obviously true and I cannot over-emphasize enough the necessity for radically changing our thinking habits, which will be discussed at greater length in a later chapter. However I must stress emphatically that I do not think it is possible to bring about the metamorphosis in our thinking, which is required, whilst not recognizing that this will only be possible if we have radically different guts in on our bellies. We develop, therefore, radically different guts in our bellies by changing our dietary habits to whole grains and vegetables and doing the ginger compress regimen.

First, it has been reasonably shown that the gradual depletion of intestinal function is induced by the gradual development of Chronic Intestinal Stagnation, which is the human organism's normal response to a staple diet of meat, eggs, refined sugar, processed, refined, chemicalized, manufactured foods etc., and this is the underlying process which leads to the development of all illnesses, both infectious and degenerative, currently known and those yet to come[2].

Thus, it seems reasonable to suggest that the restoration of intestinal integrity of function is intrinsic to any realistic attempt to the body healing itself. That is to say, clearly and certainly, any modern medicine with any pretense to being modern, which does not take as its underlying premise the natural restoration of the healthy function of the digestive/metabolic processes is doomed to failure, is medically irrelevant, and medically impertinent[3].

The essential role of the ginger compress is thus clear. I have no doubt that the doing of the ginger compresses is as necessary as changing our diet to one based on cooked whole grains and vegetables if a true and deep healing of the body is going to be at all possible. So, although the healing processes are deep mystery, we make possible our healing by doing the regimen of ginger compresses.

Another crucial insight is the symptoms of the illness process indicate the body is attempting to heal itself. The fundamental error of techno-scientific, materialistic medicine is confusing the symptoms of the illness with illness itself. It has thus directed all its efforts and human resources toward devising methods of diagnosis and eliminating symptoms, mistakenly thinking that in so doing the illnesses itself is being addressed, when, in reality, it is not. The elimination of the symptoms of illnesses, by any method, be it drug therapy, genetic therapy, radiation or surgery, means that the processes whereby the body is healing itself are suppressed, and the illness/healing process continues at a deeper level in the body.

In essence, modern medical sciences have trivialized illness and the meaning of illness. The bogus notion that anyone manifesting illness symptoms is not responsible for developing their illness simply means people are directed way from what is most important. The symptoms of illness offer profound and enormously significant lessons. Illness is a teacher for us to learn from; to learn about ourselves, to learn from the errors of commission and omission of our day-to-day lives, so we may take personal responsibility to correct our errors and heal ourselves.

And it has, I hope, not escaped the attention of the reader that eating the modern diet is a reasonably sure prescription for developing infectious and degenerative illnesses of one kind or another. In 1996[4] a report was published detailing the woeful record of modern scientific medicine in coming to grips with cancer, which confirms that this is indeed the case.

NOTES.

1. See *"Knowledge of Higher Worlds—Rudolf Steiner's Blackboard Drawings"*. (University of California, Berkeley Art Museum and Pacific Film Archives, 1997 pp. 50.).
2. What I mean by degenerative illnesses yet to come is if humanity does not find the wherewithal to change our dietary patterns to the one described here, that this, eating cooked whole grains and vegetables as our staple food, as well as changing our way of thinking, then the biological and mental-spiritual degeneration of the human race will continue apace, leading to the appearance of even more severe forms of degenerative illnesses than cancer or AIDS.
3. Rudolf Steiner, in a lecture cycle entitled *"Man as Symphony of the Creative Word"* (Rudolf Steiner Press, London, 1970, pp.182) states *"a modern system of medicine must always take the metabolic system, that is to say the normal processes of digestion, as its point of departure, and starting from there it must deduce how internal illnesses in the widest possible sense can arise from the metabolism"*. This lecture was given on November 10th, 1923 in Dornach, Switzerland.
4. February 5th 1996 issue of US News and World Report—"The War against Cancer: 26 years later." The evidence is clear—cancer is winning the war on cancer. It is no contest.

CHAPTER EIGHT

GENERAL DIETARY RECOMMENDATIONS

This chapter is intended primarily for those readers new to a macrobiotic dietary practice. Recommendations are given for anyone who wishes to support their body to heal, that is, to restore itself to vitality and well-being. A macrobiotic practice is only a diet to begin with; the diet is the main focus of our daily macrobiotic living for the first three to seven years of living our lives according to macrobiotic principles. After three to seven years of eating macrobiotically in the relatively circumspect manner described here, it will be necessary to start expanding our dietary intake to include foods, which are not discussed here. The reason this widening of diet is necessary will become apparent in the chapter on Macrobiotic Healing.

These recommendations are offered only as a guide. It must be emphasized again that any individual who decides to adopt eating these foods in the manner indicated is strongly recommended to seek out local people both knowledgeable and experienced with regards to a macrobiotic way of eating, who can offer help and advice.

There are many pitfalls to the novice to this way of eating and, although theoretically anyone can start with the appropriate books (See the chapter Getting Started and the bibliography for a list of recommended books, including cookbooks) and do well, very few appear able to do so without making mistakes.

The attentive reader will have garnered a clear picture of my feelings with regard to modern technological medicine. Nonetheless, I must emphasize that nothing written here is to be construed as having anything remotely to do with conventional medical practices or medical advice, and this book is not intended to replace conventional medical advice from a medical professional.

One major point about macrobiotic practice is it is not a medical practice; the only aspect of macrobiotic practice which it has in common with any of the many practices of medicine available today is that, in all cases, we are dealing with the human being (and with respect to modern scientific medicine, this is debatable).

It is the reality today that modern, techno-scientific, materialistic, reductionist thinking permeates every field of human endeavor. Even that of so-called Alternative and Complimentary Medicine. Thus most people today have no trouble with the idea that the human body is a machine, albeit an elaborate techno-physico-chemical complex of atoms and molecules governed by the same laws of physics and chemistry which apply in the test tube. A grotesque illusion, to be sure, a phantasm of unreality. The body of the human being (or animal or plant) is the expression of the "mineral ghost" manifesting the activity of the etheric/chi or life body of the human being, animal and plant.

Macrobiotic practice as described in this book is much wiser and more profound than any medicine yet devised by humanity because it is predicated on the spiritual reality that there is "designed into" the human organism a continuous dynamic interplay of the forces of disease and the forces of healing. It is the interplay between these two impulses that initiates the symptoms of illness as a balancing process where by the body maintains its internal balance. This is what constitutes the healing process.

Thus, the idea is to allow the appropriate dynamic balance integral to the human organism to assert itself harmoniously and to support it. This is done initially through balancing our daily eating appropriately. However, it also requires a great deal of strenuous, persistent and patient study, practice, self-reflection and purging of received prejudices, assumptions, concepts and ideas before this spiritual reality is grasped with all the implications contained in it.

Therefore it must be clearly understood that the essence of the macrobiotic way of eating has nothing to do with nutrition per se. As I have stressed repeatedly, the basis of this way of eating is yin-yang theory applied to the yin-yang make-up of the human organism. When this is done, it turns out that the appropriate dietary intake of the human being is cooked whole grains and vegetables. It is by balancing the daily intake of our food, in terms of yin and yang theory, with respect to the dynamics of the human organisms, which has determined whole grains, and vegetables are the most appropriate foods for humanity.

The question of the protein or carbohydrate or fatty acid or mineral trace element content of the food is secondary to the consideration of balancing our daily dietary intake in terms of yin and yang. It is by making the dietary intake balanced in terms of yin and yang with respect to the dynamics of the human organism that we know we will be receiving the appropriate nutrient content in the food as a consequence. This insight has of course being completely overlooked when considerations are made with regard to what is the appropriate diet for humanity from all sorts of sources. There are no magic ingredients or nutrients or substances contained in any food for these contain no healing qualities at all.

Thus when we talk about a balanced diet, which is commonplace, most people do not know what they are talking about and thus we get inundated with a vast array of "diets" containing misleading information with regard to what is the appropriate dietary balance for the human organism.

The heart of macrobiotic practice is exactly that, daily practice, and commentary on macrobiotic dietary practice by anyone who has not practiced assiduously for at least seven years and completed the three rounds of ginger compresses, is necessarily fragmentary, superficial and misleading. Macrobiotic practice is not merely an intellectual exercise.

The primary perspective in terms of macrobiotic dietary practice is qualitative rather than quantitative. As stated, the human physical organism is understood in both Traditional Oriental Medicine and Western Esotericism to be imbued with spiritual forces, which are variously called "chi", "ki" and "prana" in the East, and "etheric" forces in the West.

Food plants are also understood to be imbued and permeated with these spiritual forces. The crucial consideration in developing a mode of eating suited to the human being is to harmonize the daily dietary intake in respect of the etheric forces of the plant food we eat with the etheric dynamics of the human organism. This is accomplished by using the principles of yin and yang theory.

If this is done properly then the etheric forces of the body will gradually come into their proper balance, and this will mean that the body's physiological functions will also come into balance. Health and vitality will be the outcome of this process. Furthermore, the body will also receive all the necessary nutrients for healthy organ and tissue function.

To put it another way, by balancing the dynamics of our daily eating with the inherent dynamics of the human etheric body, we are, at the very least, not disturbing and undermining the inherent dynamics of the etheric body. This therefore allows the etheric body to assert its proper dynamic homeostasis. At best, in eating this way, we are actively supporting the inherent dynamic balance of the etheric body. This means the our body will heal itself and maintain its health and vitality

General considerations.

All foods eaten are cultivated organically or bio-dynamically, where possible.

Foods eaten are cultivated locally and eaten in season.

Foods are prepared in their whole form; for example, we start with the whole carrot, wash it, cut it appropriately and cook it.

Consume meals consisting of a variety of color.

Vary our meals using different grains, vegetables, beans and condiments.

Avoid using aluminum cookware, coated cookware and microwave ovens.

Eliminate, by and large to begin with, consuming refined, frozen, packaged and canned foods, and animal protein in any form (including all dairy foods), fruit, refined sugar, refined flour products, as well as drugs and alcohol and any foods which contain additives(preservatives, emulsifiers, vitamins, artificial colors, dyes, "natural flavors" etc.).

Chew the food well, meaning take small mouthfuls, chewing each mouthful at least 20-30 times, and chew quickly.

Do not overeat. It is best to leave the table after eating your meal feeling like you could eat a little bit more. Do not eat any food within three hours of going to bed at night.

Foods available for human consumption can be categorized into four different groups.

Primary Food—Whole Cereal Grains.

Whole grains are considered the staple food for the human being and have been since the dawn of recorded history. Over the course of the day, approximately half of our daily consumption is comprised of cooked whole grains[1]. Whole grains include brown rice, wheat, barley, oats, rye, buckwheat, millet, corn, teff, amaranth and quinoa.[1]

Also, always cook whole grains with a small amount of sea salt. The suggestion that cooking is necessary is somewhat controversial these days. However, there are very sound reasons for cooking our food and these include:

1. Cooking is a stage of "pre-digestion" in that it prepares the food for proper digestion and assimilation.
2. The human digestive system is not "designed" to digest raw vegetable matter properly.

3. Raw foods compared to cooked foods have a cooling effect upon the body. If all the illnesses of humanity are classified into two groups, those resulting from too much heat in the body or those resulting from too much cold, then all degenerative illnesses fall into the latter category.
4. From yin-yang theory, raw foods are more yin than cooked foods. This is not to say we can never eat raw foods but their appropriateness is usually limited to hot climates, seasons or on hot days and when our condition allows.

Secondary Foods—Vegetables,

Vegetables are cooked, and least half of our daily intake of vegetables must be steamed or boiled leafy greens. The remainder of the vegetables may be cooked in a wide variety of ways, such as steamed, sautéed in olive or sesame oil, boiled, or baked, etc.

Supplementary Foods—Beans and Sea Vegetables.

Beans are not actually necessary as a daily food, however, most people changing over to a macrobiotic dietary regimen come from a diet heavy in animal protein, and will find it easier to maintain their macrobiotic practice by eating cooked beans for the first two to three years.

For regular use adzuki beans, chickpeas and lentils are recommended. Other beans can be used occasionally. I am personally a strong critic of tofu (soybean curd), feeling it is a very detrimental food and only to be used on an occasional basis and then only in small amounts. The reason I think it is detrimental to eat is it is a highly refined food; so eating it is like eating refined white flour. Also it is too high in protein and fat content.

Seaweeds, such as kombu, dulse, kelp, sea palm, wakame, hijiki, arame, mekabu and nori can be prepared in a variety of ways. They can be cooked with grains, beans and vegetables, and used in soups and side dishes. It is recommended they be eaten daily in small quantities.

Small amounts of white meat fish; shellfish can be eaten occasionally if our condition allows, once or twice a week.

Cooked fruit desserts, as well as fresh fruits and dried fruits, may be eaten occasionally depending on our condition. Only locally grown fruit of temperate climate origin if we live in a temperate climate. Tropical and semi-tropical fruit is only eaten if we live in those climates. Fruit and vegetable juices are generally avoided except during the hot summer months, when we eat raw salads, again depending on our physical condition. Cooked nuts and seeds maybe consumed in small amounts as a snack or garnish.

Foods For Pleasure.

These include any food available for human consumption not mentioned above. They are only to be eaten if we are in good health. If we are in poor health or have any type of degenerative condition, it is generally recommended to avoid this category of food. None of them are necessary. Some examples include any form of meat, dairy food, alcohol, refined flour products, sugar in any form, soft drinks and eggs.

Soups.

It is highly recommended for at least the first three to seven years of our macrobiotic practice to consume one bowl of miso soup every day. The soup is made with vegetables and sea vegetables and sometimes beans, to which miso, a fermented soybean paste, is added.

Beverages.

Total liquid intake (not including soup) is limited to between three and five eight-ounce glasses per day. Of course, if we are thirsty, we can drink more than the recommended amount. Beverages recommended include spring water, purified tap water, roasted barley tea, roasted bancha twig tea, and dried burdock root tea, dried dandelion root tea and grain coffee.

NUTRITIONAL CONSIDERATIONS.

A vast amount of research has being conducted over the past sixty years, and especially the past ten to twenty years, to determine the important and essential nutrients the human physical organism needs for optimum daily functioning. This has led to the present concern over nutrient deficiencies in various diets.

It is perhaps stating the obvious that the modern diet is almost entirely nutrient poor, and thus people are exhorted to ingest all kinds of nutrient supplements, including vitamins, trace elements, minerals, enzymes, etc., in one form or other. (The industry had sales of 11 billion dollars in 2001).

There are three main points to consider with regard to this problem. Firstly, because most people eat a diet based in what is available on the supermarket shelf, most of these foods are manufactured and processed foods, meaning they are denatured, devitalized and refined, etc., they therefore tend to be nutrient deficient.

Secondly, even if our diet is nutrient adequate, the presence of Chronic Intestinal Stagnation in the small intestine assures these nutrients will not be assimilated properly, which means people are continuously undernourished. Consequently people feel hungry all the time, overeat, and eat more refined foods more often, which are easier to assimilate, leading to the widespread problem of obesity.

Thirdly, and this is a major problem which is not recognized by modern scientific research at all, is considerations of the quality of the vitamins, trace elements, and minerals and so forth, that are being ingested. We may be ingesting all the vitamins, trace elements and minerals the body needs but if the are "qualitatively insufficient" then they are not being ingested by the body in a form the body can assimilate and utilize properly.

The proper activity of the nutrients in the body, contained in the food we eat every day, I refer to as their "accurate or inaccurate biological (spiritual) activity". Their functional accuracy or inaccuracy is contingent on the form in which they are being ingested.

Since all minerals, vitamins, etc., present in the brown rice, barley, carrot, kale, broccoli, etc. are embedded in what may be called a "natural matrix" in the whole grain or vegetable, their proper, accurate, biological (spiritual) activity in the human organism is the effect of their own particular form, as well as the context of the "natural matrix", in which they are embedded in the whole food.

Thus, if a vitamin, mineral, etc., is extracted or processed in any way from its natural source, or, more seriously, synthesized, the substance thus extracted, processed and manufactured bears little resemblance to the vitamins, trace elements and minerals found in their natural form in the whole food. *"Chemical foods are not the same as the those provided by nature, even if they have the same constituents²"*. In other words, a Vitamin C molecule extracted from kale looked at through a microscope may be identical to a synthetic Vitamin C looked at through a microscope, but the fact is they are not the same substance. That is to say the functional biological (spiritual) integrity of the activity of any nutrient is not only a function of their particular form, but is also contingent on the natural matrix in which they are found in their natural state in the whole grain or vegetable.

If people who have a healthy digestive system ingest these unnatural, synthetic, artificial vitamin, mineral and other supplements, which are easily recognized by the fact that they are purchased in pill, powder or potion form, or as additives in a host of food products, the process of assimilation will result in these supplements being "screened out" by the healthy mucous epithelial lining of a healthy digestive tract.

If you recall, I mentioned earlier that the mucous epithelial lining of the intestinal tract acts an "inverted tongue", which, when it "tastes" these unnatural substances, rejects them just as you would spit out something you found distasteful in your mouth.

If, on the other hand, the digestive tract has Chronic Intestinal Stagnation, then necessarily its functions are compromised, and these unnatural substances will likely be assimilated, and whatever their effect it will not be their proper accurate biological (spiritual) activity. Furthermore, in the massive doses in which they are consumed it is highly likely they will have toxic effects upon the body's immune functions[3].

Bearing this mind, analysis of the wide variety of whole grains, vegetables, beans and sea vegetables consumed in a macrobiotic dietary practice shows these foods are nutrient rich. Nevertheless it may be helpful to address the commonly held misconception that a macrobiotic dietary practice is deficient in certain nutrients. Of primary concern are protein, vitamin C, (ascorbic acid), vitamin B2 (riboflavin), vitamin B12, vitamin A, calcium, iron and caloric energy.

Protein.

It is a commonly held misconception that a predominantly vegetarian diet is protein deficient. In truth, even purely vegetarian diets (diets containing no animal protein at all) are not protein deficient, and one can get all the essential amino acids from eating vegetables alone. Vegetable protein is qualitatively superior to animal protein, as it does not contain saturated fats associated with cancer and heart disease. Another important point is the amount of daily protein intake generally recommended is grossly in excess of what we actually need. The adequate daily intake for the average active adult is merely one ounce (28.6 grams) of protein[4].

Vitamin C.

A half cup of kale meets the US recommended daily amount (RDA) of 16 milligrams a day. In fact, leafy green vegetables contain larger amounts of Vitamin C than an equal serving of citrus fruits, with broccoli, brussel sprouts, and kale containing twice as much.

Vitamin B2 (riboflavin).

The concern that vitamin B2 may be lacking in vegetable diets is based on the misconception that riboflavin is only available in dairy foods. In fact, kale and mustard greens contain as much B2 as dairy food. US RDA is 0.57 milligrams per 1000 calories of food consumed.

Vitamin B12.

The concerns of a deficiency of vitamin B12 stem from a misconception that is only available from animal sources. In fact vitamin B12 is present in more than adequate amounts in fermented foods such as miso, soy sauce, tamari and in sea vegetables[5].

Vitamin A.

Vitamin A is plentiful in many vegetables.

Calcium.

Per cup serving, steamed leafy greens supply as much calcium (as well vitamin B2 and iron) as cow's milk, if not more. Also, sea vegetables, which are recommended to be consumed daily, contain astonishing amounts of calcium.

Interestingly, osteoporosis (weakening of the bones), often thought to be primarily due to calcium deficiency, is relatively common in the industrially developed countries, whereas its occurrence is much less frequent in less developed countries where dairy foods are not widely consumed. The World Health Organization considers average daily calcium intake of 400-500 milligrams adequate.

Iron.

To maintain healthy quality blood, adequate sources of iron are needed for the formation of red blood cells. Iron is plentiful in many grains and vegetables.

Vitamin D.

The problem of vitamin D deficiency is averted if individuals eat a wide variety of grains and vegetables, including small amounts of fermented foods such as miso and macrobiotic style pickled foods like sauerkraut, dill pickles etc., and get enough sunshine.

Caloric energy.

There is plenty of caloric energy in a whole grain and vegetable diet. Many people experience a remarkable increase in their level of vitality and stamina when adopting a macrobiotic dietary program, which is, according to the caloric energy requirements generally regarded as adequate for the average adult, hopelessly inadequate.

Whole grains, which are emphasized here as being the primary food for the human being, are widely recognized as being nutrient rich. Paul Mangelsdorf, writing in the July 1963 issue of Scientific American states, "*cereal grains . . .represent a 5-in-1 food supply which contains complex carbohydrates, proteins, fat, minerals and vitamins. A whole cereal grain, if its food value is not destroyed by the over-refinement of modern methods of food processing, come closer than any other plant for providing an adequate diet.*"[6]

NOTES.

1. The actual daily proportion of whole grains for any person depends on many factors including age, body type, health condition, lifestyle and habitat with respect to climate, the season, weather patterns, geography and altitude.
2. Rudolf Steiner in his lecture cycle, "*The Fall of The Spirits of Darkness*", Chapter 2, page 29. (Rudolf Steiner Press, London, 1993.).
3. This is beginning to be recognized by the scientific community—see New York Times, April 9th 1998; "*study finds possible harm from higher doses of vitamin C*", by Jane Brody. Also Arizona Republic, May 2 1996, printing a story from a Minneapolis St. Paul Star Tribune "*Eat your fruits and vegetables, study says supplements futile.*" by Gordon Slovuts.
4. See the chapter on protein in "*The Essentials Of Nutrition*" by Dr. Gerhardt Schmidt M.D., published by Biodynamic Literature.
5. A major source of vitamin B12 is the human appendix (see "*The Dynamics of Nutrition*" by Dr. Gerhardt Schmidt M.D., published by Biodynamic Literature). Microorganisms living in the appendix produce B vitamins (including B12) as well as assist in their assimilation. An important food which stimulates the life cycle of these organisms is whole grain sourdough bread, so it is important to eat two to three slices of this a day as part of one's daily grain intake.
6. In the chapter on Blood Alchemy I discuss the theory of transformation of food into red blood cells and mentioned the transmutation of magnesium into iron during the process of transformation of chlorophyll into hemoglobin. Theoretically, in a healthy human being with no Chronic Intestinal Stagnation, it is possible to regard the human organism as an "alchemical vessel" which can create any substance it needs according to its needs at any one instant. For example, enzymes, vitamins etc., provided the body is receiving cooked whole grains and vegetables as its main food source.

CHAPTER NINE

PRINCIPLES OF YIN AND YANG

Anyone starting a macrobiotic dietary practice without studying yin and yang can do so adequately, experiencing increasing health benefits physically, emotionally and mentally, for only a certain period of time, perhaps three to five years at the most. However, since a macrobiotic dietary practice is not dieting in the conventional sense, if we have not studied and begun to understand the principles, which inform our practice, principally yin-yang theory and its derivative, the Five Transformation Theory, we will find that around the three to five year range, our practice will get "bogged down". As George Ohsawa stated it, "a theory without a practice is useless, a practice without a theory is dangerous".

It is commonplace for people to have started on a macrobiotic dietary practice and given up after two to three years of so; one constantly hears people saying "Oh yes, I tried macrobiotics for a while back in." whatever decade they happened to have tried it. The number of people, who have started a macrobiotic practice and given up after two to three years, or less, is probably 80%.

There are many reasons for this phenomenon, and I feel one of the most important to be the lack of study of yin-yang theory. The result is that people do not know how or when, by and large, to make the necessary adjustments to their macrobiotic practice as their condition improves. People also tend to have the general misunderstanding that it is a diet when it is not. The fact it is not a diet necessarily means we have to make adjustments as we go along after we have been doing the more restricted regimen for two to three years.

These dietary adjustments generally mean we have to start widening the choices of food available to us, so we can eventually eat any food we want, all the while maintaining our daily staple intake of cooked whole grains and vegetables. In actual fact, it is not in accord with the macrobiotic philosophy for anyone to consume the same dietary intake from season to season, year in and year out; a dietary intake suitable for a person in a certain condition is not appropriate as their condition improves.

Another very important reason to learn to understand yin-yang theory is to change our way of thinking. This is of paramount importance because we cannot heal ourselves unless we change our habitual mode of thinking. The presently dominant mode of thinking in the world can be characterized as scientific, materialistic, reductionist thinking, which has developed over the past 400 years. And it is this manner of thinking which everybody has as their habitual mode of thinking, whether they are aware of it or not.

This manner of thinking has arisen from the study of the material natural world, its basis for knowledge being the world of minerals and chemicals. From exhaustive studies, experimentation and observation of phenomena of the mineral kingdom have been derived the laws of physics and chemistry. These chemical and physical laws have then been applied in the manipulation of matter, thereby developing a very clever and in many instances, beneficial material technology. This is fine as long as the chemical and physical laws are understood to be pertinent and applicable only to chemicals and minerals.

However, this mode of thinking I characterize as materialistic—scientific—reductionist, permeates every branch of knowledge and learning, and most human endeavors, today. We need to wake up to the fact we are totally deluded if we think the plant, the animal and the human being is merely a more elaborate and complex arrangements of physics and chemistry than is a rock or stone. In other words, it is not logically possible to derive true understanding and knowledge of living organisms by means of the laws of physics and chemistry.

The world is suffering grievously under the burden of this delusion. It is not an exaggeration to say all of problems the world is now experiencing (and has been for several decades), be they ecological, environmental, economic, legal, social, political, medical, educational or religious—are the result of the predominant mode thinking characterized as scientific—materialistic—reductionist. It is therefore fairly obvious to draw the conclusion that this mode of thinking will not help us in solving any of these problems. In fact, solutions to present problems are clearly not possible by means of this way of thinking. This is why the problems have so far proven to be intractable and have gotten worse.

We therefore need to develop a radically different way of thinking which has its epistemology based on the logically undeniable fact that the worlds of plants, animals, and human beings, and, in the final analysis, even the world of minerals, are the expression, the manifestations and symptoms of laws operating in the world of the spirit, the world which creates, imbues and permeates the physical world.

Rudolf Steiner states that the development of the intellectual capacity of the human soul so we could objectively investigate the natural, material world and develop the capacity to think independently, out of our own resources of the soul, beginning around 1413 A.D., was a necessary step in the evolutionary development of human consciousness. However, any human being taking the materialistic, scientific world—view to its logical conclusion cannot but admit it is not possible to find in it any real satisfaction for the soul, by this means, as to why the phenomena of the world and nature function the way they do.

Thus, having a reached the necessary "brick wall" at the end of scientific materialism, we must posit an invisible domain, lying behind the veil of the physical senses, which is behind/within the material phenomena and is the fundamental cause of all phenomena—mineral, plant, animal and human—in the realm of the physical world behaving the way they do. This is the world/s of spiritual beings, forces and activities. It is the tragedy of modern scientific materialism that is has no understanding of the physical worlds of minerals, plants, animals and human beings. The reality is that all physical phenomena perceived by the physical sense organs are both the expression of and vehicle for a wide variety of spiritual impulses—the tragedy of modern science is that it only sees the physical object, and denies the spiritual forces giving rise to it.

The fact that people inhabiting the world today do not find this logical conclusion, that the physical world is an expression and vehicle for the action of spiritual forces directed by the activities of spiritual beings, admissible, is more a statement about humanity's present enthrallment with the delusion of modern scientific materialism, feebleness of soul, intellectual cowardice and less than stringent, accurate scientific observation of material phenomena, than it is about the truthfulness of the logical conclusion itself[1].

As a first step, or bridge, towards developing this radically different way of thinking, the study and understanding of yin and yang is very helpful, because it is predicated on the knowledge of hidden (that is, imperceptible by the physical sense organs) forces and dynamics lying within and behind material phenomena which give them their form and dynamic of function and activity. Yin and yang is a "descriptive language" to help us understand the dynamics of spiritual activity. Since understanding yin and yang is radically different from the conventional habit of scientific materialistic reductionist thinking, it requires a rigorous and consistent retraining of our own thinking[2].

It is also very important to realize developing our understanding of yin and yang is as necessary to our healing as is eating cooked whole grains and vegetables. In fact is entirely doubtful developing our physical, emotional, mental and spiritual health and vitality is possible without radically changing our way of thinking in the manner described here, no matter how well we are eating. The necessity of developing our understanding of yin and yang is essential as it is not an intellectual arrangement, it can never be understood from a purely intellectual standpoint. For, although on the surface yin and yang appear to be simplicity itself, and in a certain respect it is, it is also complex, profound and subtle[3].

One problem, which I have already alluded to, is anyone coming to this book with any sort of tradition or background in Traditional Chinese Medicine, may look at the description of the yin and yang qualities, attributes and tendencies that follows and conclude the macrobiotic understanding of yin and yang is in error. And indeed it is, from the perspective of Traditional Chinese Medicine. However, George Ohsawa, who I refer to as the "re-discoverer" of macrobiotic principles and practices, asserts that the one he elaborated on is the original one and the metaphysical one of Traditional Chinese Medicine is a later development.

In essence, if we study the *I Ching* or Book Of Change, which is the consummate expression of yin and yang philosophy from the Chinese perspective, it states that "heaven", being the generator of all things, is more creative, active, dynamic and is therefore more yang than the expression of its creative activity, which is called "earth". "Earth", which is, in contrast to "heaven", more passive, receptive, and still, is therefore more yin than "heaven". In the I Ching "heaven" is called Great Yang and "earth" is called Great Yin.

George Ohsawa said that on the other hand, from the perspective of an individual living on the earth, that heaven is a wide, vast, relatively empty expanse flung out above us and is therefore more yin relative to the earth, which is from this perspective, a solid, compacted, physical object, floating in the wide expanse of space. It is therefore more yang than space or "heaven". From this different perspective George Ohsawa developed yin-yang theory as presented here.

Thus, neither one is incorrect as long as they are not mixed up; if we are consistent in our interpretations from each perspective, then we will not make errors, excepting those made because of our lack of understanding of whichever interpretation of yin and yang we are using. There's no reason one cannot learn both; however, my advice is if we intend to start a macrobiotic dietary practice is to study the explanation given here. We need to devote at least an hour day to this study until we begin to develop our understanding very well, before studying Traditional Chinese Medicine's interpretation of yin and yang. This is at least a 2-3 year proposition, while simultaneously adopting a macrobiotic dietary program, which is one of the applications of yin-yang theory, and therefore a great way to study it is to learn to cook macrobiotically.

The Principles of Yin and Yang.

1. Oneness, God, the ineffable creative continuously manifests two tendencies of dynamic spiritual activity, which are in all places and times under the continuous guidance of the One. Together, these three manifests the "ten thousand things"; that is, all visible and invisible phenomena of the relative world.
2. The two tendencies are called yin, centrifugality and yang, centripitality.
3. Yin attracts yang; yang attracts yin.
4. Yang repels yang; yin repels yin
5. At their extremes of movement, extreme yin changes into or creates yang: likewise, extreme yang changes into or creates yin.
6. The greater the polarity between yin and yang, the greater the force of attraction between them. The more alike two phenomena are in terms of yin and yang, the greater the force of repulsion between them.
7. Yin and yang are constantly changing into one another.
8. No phenomenon is completely, absolutely yang or completely, absolutely yin. All phenomena are permeated with both yin and yang tendencies.
9. No phenomenon is neutral, that is perfectly balanced. Yin or yang is present in excess relative to one another in all phenomena at one time or another in continuous dynamic interplay.
10. Under the guidance of the One, all inter-relationships of yin and yang are always tending toward harmony,

The Ten Principles of Yin and Yang are, so to speak, the rules of the game. In addition to learning these by heart, we also need to learn what I call the ABC's of yin and yang also.

These are the properties, attributes and tendencies of Yin and Yang as follows:

Properties, Attributes and Tendencies of YIN and YANG.

	YIN	YANG
	(Centrifugal)	(Centripetal)
Tendency	Expansion	Contraction
	Diffusion	Fusion
	Dissipation	Organization
	Dispersion	Assimilation
	Separation	Gathering
	Decomposition	Composition

	Disintegration	Integration
Direction	Upward	Downward
	Outward	Inward
	Horizontally, beneath ground	Horizontally, above ground
	Ascent and vertical	Descent and horizontal
Movement	More inactive and slower	More active and faster
Vibration	Shorter wave & Higher frequency	Longer wave & Lower frequency

Light	Darker	Brighter
Diurnal Rhythm	Night	Day
Seasons	Winter	Summer
Temperature	Colder	Hotter
Texture	Rougher	Smoother
Density	Softer	Harder
Weight	Lighter	Heavier
Moisture	Wetter	Drier
Height	Taller	Shorter
Size	Larger	Smaller

Color	Violet Indigo Blue Green	Yellow Orange Red
Elements	N, O, K, P, Ca, etc.	H, C, Na, As, Mg, etc.
Climatic effects	Tropical Climate	Colder Climate
Sex	Female	Male
Heavenly Bodies	Moon	Sun
Biological Kingdom	Animal	Vegetable
Organ Structure	More hollow & expansive	More compacted and condensed
Nerves	More peripheral, sympathetic	More central, parasympathetic
Attitude	More gentle, negative	More assertive, positive
Work	More psychological & mental	More physical and social
Dimension	Space	Time

This is by no means an exhaustive list, and by learning it you can add many more in observing the world around you using yin and yang thinking.

NOTES.

1. The whole of Rudolf Steiner's life and work was dedicated to giving the world the basis and means for understanding and perceiving the world of spirit and how it relates to the physical world. There are over 450 volumes of his books, lectures, poems, sketches, drawings, etc., available (not all in English translations yet), and I list the basic ones in the bibliography.

2. In my case, and admittedly I am slow of learning, it was only after the first three years of daily study of yin and yang while adopting my macrobiotic dietary practice, that I began to get the first glimmer of understanding yin and yang. The higher our level of learning, in the conventional sense, the more difficult it is to retrain our thinking processes in order to understand yin and yang.

3. It is as well to note here that yin and yang are not the names of deities, have no creative powers and have nothing to do with good and evil. In fact, no moral attributes are associated with them.

Chapter Ten

ON THE WAY OF A MACROBIOTIC DIETARY PRACTICE

This chapter is written for those readers who have decided to adopt a macrobiotic dietary practice, to give an idea of what to expect during the healing process.

The most important point to understand is why anyone would undertake a macrobiotic dietary practice. It is not to cure any illness, and it should be clear, if what I have written thus far has been understood, that there is no cure for any illness. So if a cure is what you're looking for, there are thousands of cures, miracle cures, wonder drugs, new—age super foods, genetic therapies, regenerative medicine, and the like being heavily promoted in the world, and, no doubt, you can find what you are looking for in that realm, if that is what you want.

The macrobiotic characterization of any symptoms that a person may be experiencing is these symptoms indicate that the person is "out-of-balance" in relation to the rhythmical, dynamic order of nature and the cosmos, not only with respect to our eating habits, but also our feelings, way of thinking, and attitudes, world-view, work, moral character, relationships with other people, family life, etc. This is really the one and only dis-ease, universal to all human beings, and all the illness syndromes, which have been experienced by humanity, are the symptomology of this one dis-ease.

The individual is responsible for developing the illness symptoms he or she is manifesting, and is therefore the only one who can heal him or herself, as described here. As "balance with nature and the cosmos" is gradually restored, the symptoms indicating to us that we are "out-of-balance" disappear; that is, we heal ourselves.

The fundamental purpose for adopting a macrobiotic practice and lifestyle is to change the present, self-destructive course of world events by taking personal responsibility for creating a radically different, healthy and constructive culture and civilization.

It is clear the present world culture, based, as it is on materialistic, scientific reductionist thinking, and the "technological imperative" that is the driving force behind this thinking, is a sick world culture. If we observe the world and the people inhabiting it, as one organism, all current events, be they social, ecological, environmental, economic, medical, political, education, etc., are symptoms of a profoundly ill and decrepit organism. There is no need to point out all the symptoms as you can readily observe them for yourselves every day in the newspapers and magazines, on television, walking on the street and, closer to home, in your families.

The symptoms of illness of the world culture indicate the world organism is attempting to heal itself. However, like the human physical organism when it is manifesting symptoms of a sick life, if we do not so order our personal disharmony and imbalanced way of life by changing our way of eating, thinking, feeling and actions to support and, harmonize ourselves with the body's healing forces, then the body becomes sicker and sicker. So it is for the world organism, which has no prospect of becoming healthy unless we see that all the events going on in the world are the symptoms, writ large, of our own individual dis-harmony and sickness.

Thus, the world is facing no prospect other than to fall into its own graveyard, which we are digging every day with the shovel of techno-scientific materialistic thinking, as long as we think the problems of the world can be solved by means of legal, political, economic or military strategies The only realistic solution is to act on, each and every one of us, the reality that we are personally responsible for the destiny of the earth. We take this responsibility in hand by undertaking the task of healing ourselves. I've mentioned the importance of karma, in our personal lives: karma also applies to society and the world; that is, there is also social and world karma.

With regard to karma, we each realize the conditions prevailing on the earth today are largely resulting from our moral and immoral thoughts, words and actions in our past lives. Thus, by consciously taking personal responsibility for healing ourselves we are also consciously preparing for both our life in the spirit world between death and rebirth as well as preparing for our next incarnation on the earth[1].

This is an inspiring prospect, worthy of the tremendously arduous, patient and sincere, consistent and disciplined effort which is required, and the beginning step is to adopt a macrobiotic dietary practice and the regimen of ginger compresses. Along with studying yin and yang.

In order to understand the process of healing ourselves it is helpful to look at the stages of development of eating macrobiotically. As mentioned there are seven levels of judgment, where judgment means developing the ability of discernment in evaluating any phenomena. These levels of judgment can be applied to any human activity, and here they are applied to the process of eating macrobiotically.

Mechanical.

At the beginning of our macrobiotic practice there is a justifiable feeling of being overwhelmed and confused by all the new terminology, new foods etc. At this stage we really have no idea what we are doing. The essential first step is to start learning how to cook macrobiotically, so we obtain one or two macrobiotic cookbooks, purchase the necessary supplies and any utensils we may need that we do not already have in our kitchen.

And right here we come across a major error, which many people make when beginning a macrobiotic practice. It cannot be emphasized enough how essential to our healing is learning the art of cooking macrobiotically. The widespread practice of finding someone to cook our meals for us means, fundamentally, that we are less than sincere about wanting to heal ourselves.

The attitude here is macrobiotic food and the way it is cooked is some kind of panacea for all ills and sicknesses. This is an extension of the "pill" or "magic bullet" mentality, which is all-pervasive today. It also appears that the medical scientific community has this chronic illness that makes people think that there is some kind of magic bullet the will solve the problem of all the illnesses of humanity. The fact is there is no substance of any kind a human being can take into his or her body that can heal it. The effort taken to learn how to prepare and cook our macrobiotic meals is the foundation for our body to begin and maintain its healing process.

At the mechanical level our aim is to get the recommended macrobiotic foods into our bodies as best as we know how, using a macrobiotic cookbook as well as taking as many cooking classes as is necessary, if it all possible. As time goes by, our cooking skills will gradually improve.

Sensory.

The significance of this level is the food we cook tastes nourishing and delicious. The difficulty can arise here for many people in that when we first start cooking macrobiotically, the resulting cooked whole grains and vegetables do not have much of a taste, being somewhat dull and bland[2]. However, the fault does not lie in the food, but in our taste buds.

As a result of longtime consumption of the high fat, salt and sugar content of the modern diet, not to mention all the spices and "enriched" foods in it, our taste buds have been bludgeoned into insensitivity. Thus, the subtle taste of the unalloyed cooked whole grains and vegetables eludes, to begin with, our dulled sense of taste. However, after a few weeks of eating these foods, and chewing them thoroughly, our taste buds recover their sensitivity and the food begins to taste delicious.

Emotional.

As we continue cooking and eating these foods, the basis of which is harmonizing ourselves with the earth, nature and the cosmos, a time comes when we begin to feel our body has a definite sense of "being at home with itself" for the first time in many a long year. A subtle feeling of bodily comfort and lightness pervades the sensibilities, and the realization arrives, at least it did for me, that I am meant to be here on earth at this particular time.

This in stark contrast to the dauntingly meaningless and nihilistically delusional fable on the origins of human life, of why and how we are living on the earth, sanctimoniously spun together by modern materialistic science, with its usual banal and absurd hubris.

I felt not only connected with the earthly and the cosmic, I also felt my life, no matter how insignificant it may be in the worldly sense, had meaning for both heaven and earth. This was an actual feeling, not something of an idle thought or fantasy, and took me by surprise. Consequently, as this feeling/perception gradually settled into my psyche, it lifted my spirits considerably, and I developed a great strengthening of inner confidence, fidelity, which continues to this day.

Intellectual.

As we continue our practice, we reach the stage where it is necessary to apply ourselves to learning and understanding the principles of macrobiotic practice and living, imbibing and digesting its theoretical underpinnings in all its simplicity **and** complexity. It is important to realize that any macrobiotic practice is not a diet per se; it is a manner of living, which includes a dietary practice, which changes according to our changing condition, and circumstances of living.

The beginning of a macrobiotically informed way of living places a strong emphasis on a macrobiotic dietary practice which is well demarcated, circumscribed, and delineated, but is not intended, nor is it healthy, to be eating the same way for years on end. If we do make the mistake of eating the same way year in and year out we actually end up worse off, physically, emotionally, mentally and spiritually, than when we started.

Thus, we need to apply ourselves diligently and perseveringly to the study of yin-yang theory. We study yin and yang not only to apply it to the proper selection, preparation and cooking our food on a daily and seasonal basis, taking into account our changing condition as we go along; we also study yin and yang in order to change our way of thinking. Another important tool in macrobiotic practice we need to learn and understand is the Five Transformation Theory.

As I have already mentioned, it took me my first three and one half years of macrobiotic practice to begin to get a glimmer of understanding of yin and yang. There are two main reasons why yin and yang are hard to grasp, the most important being our state of health because this determines our clarity of thinking. If we are in poor condition, which most of us are to begin with, then our thinking tends to be unclear, confused, scattered and cloudy. It is only as our condition starts to improve (while adopting our macrobiotic dietary program while we are studying yin and yang) that yin and yang become more clearly understood.

The other main reason it is modern education. The more educated we are, the more difficult it is to understand yin and yang, as yin and yang thinking is radically different from conventional thinking. Thus the higher we go in terms of modern education from grade school to university the more difficult it is to understand yin and yang.

Social.

At this stage we begin to recognize the social[3] ramifications of our dietary[4] choices on one hand and, on the other, we begin to realize that if we wish to experience continued improvement in our emotional, mental and physical condition, we need to start sharing what we have learned and experienced with whomever we find receptive, including family members, friends, colleagues, etc., for a healthy macrobiotic practice is very difficult, if not impossible, when we are isolated.

This can be done in any way we find fitting, simply by buying a friend a macrobiotic book, talking about it, hosting potlucks, and going on to giving cooking classes, lectures and offering counseling.

A word of caution; many people get so caught up in their enthusiasm as they begin to feel the manifold benefits of adopting their macrobiotic practice, they begin to teach before they are really ready. It is better to study for several years, either by taking classes in the various macrobiotic institutions where we can learn more formally about macrobiotic philosophy and practice or study informally with an experienced practitioner, before we start doing any teaching, simply because it takes this long before we gain sufficient experience to be able to teach.

To delineate and follow the threads of the positive effects of a macrobiotic life socially, economically and politically as well as the ramifications and implications of a significant number of people adopting a macrobiotic manner of living is beyond the scope of this book. It would require another book to be able to follow through and describe all these but you can use your own mind and imagination to be able to see these for yourself in following these threads, if you carry out the exercise.

Religious.

At this stage the recognition develops that we use our macrobiotic dietary practice in order to aid and support our spiritual development. Many of the world's religions and esoteric schools had, and have, many admonitions and instructions about what to eat, what not to eat, when to eat, how to eat etc. These practices were and are based on a deep knowledge of foods which are of benefit for spiritual development and which are hindrances[5].

Supreme.

At this stage our daily dietary habits are completely free of any constraints and any food is eaten with no compulsion to choose one over the other so we eat any food we want with great joy and gratitude, and we do not get sick.

This statement usually elicits a gasp of incredulity when I make it at various macrobiotic lectures and workshops I give. People do not appear to believe me when I say this, but the fact is a macrobiotic life is one, which is fundamentally about being a free and independent human being.

Actually, the idea that we get to the stage in our macrobiotic practice where we can eat anything we want should not come as a shock to anyone who has been studying macrobiotic literature to any extent. It has been a fundamental teaching of macrobiotic practice for at least fifty years. George Ohsawa (1891-1966), widely regarded as the principle initiator of macrobiotic practice and philosophy in modern times, wrote in his book Guidebook for Living,

> *"Whereas long ago I could not smoke or drink, I can do either as I like. I enjoy any cuisine . . .Western, Chinese, Japanese or Indian. I like fruit, candy, chocolate, and whiskey very much. If I choose to use these things now, I am able to avoid harm because I can balance yin and yang.*

I tell you this because many people think that macrobiotics is a 20th century variety of stoicism. **But he who cannot drink, smoke, eat fruit or meat is a cripple.** *Macrobiotics is a way to build health that enables us to eat anything we like without being obsessed or driven to do so. Macrobiotics is not a negative way of living . . .it is positive, creative, artistic, religious, philosophical" (his emphasis[6]).*

In the case of Rudolf Steiner (1861-1925) on discussing whether a person becomes what they eat or not, remarks, *"Man can nourish himself in such a fashion that he undermines his invisible independence. In so doing he makes himself the expression of what he eats. Yet he ought to nourish himself in such a manner that he becomes less the slave of his nutritional habits. Here spiritual science can direct him. The wrong food can easily transform us into what we eat, but by permeating ourselves with knowledge of the spiritual life, we can strive to become free and independent, then the food we eat will not hinder us from achieving the full potential of what we, as man, ought to be."[7]*

I have repeated several times in the course of this writing the statement there is nothing we can take in which can cure us of any illness, there is no cure for any illness, there has never been, nor will there be any cure for any of the illnesses and afflictions of the human organism, nor is the finding of a cure even desirable, if it were at all possible.

Now, the opposite statement is also correct; there is nothing in and of itself that we can ingest, in the normal course of daily life, which is the sole cause of any illness. Clearly, I do not mean if we consume six ounces of arsenic, or large doses of lead or mercury, or carbon monoxide, we are not going to experience illness or even death. What I am driving at is any symptomology, any constellation of symptoms, signifies our habits of daily living, including eating, thinking and feeling, are not in harmony with our place of habitation on earth or the spiritual realities of the cosmos.

The human organism is a microcosmic expression in the physical plane of the entire cosmos. When we look around us and observe plants and animals in all their variety and profusion, and observe the material expression of the spiritual cosmos in, for example, the orbit of the moon around the earth every twenty eight days or so, the orderly passage of the diurnal rhythm every 24 hours as the earth turns on its axis, the passage of the four seasons as the earth circles the sun every three hundred and sixty four and a quarter days, in unfailing sequence year after year, this observation gives us the feeling the physical cosmos and nature are informed by and permeated with a profoundly harmonious wisdom.

Thus, if we can discern the laws and principles of this wisdom, which underlies natural and cosmic harmony, and shape our lives accordingly, we will therefore be consciously harmonizing our lives with of the earth and the cosmos. This idea is fundamental to macrobiotic practice and living translated into statement that health, in the sense discussed in the introduction, is a condition arising out of consciously living in an accord with "the order of the universe", both naturally and spiritually.

Clearly this is not a new idea. It lies behind all pagan cultures, it is central to all Far Eastern religious traditions, it is found in Celtic, Greek, Egyptian and Hebrew cultures, as well as in ancient South American cultures like the Aztecs and Mayan, as well as the Hopis, etc.

It is also a central (if completely overlooked) tenet, simply because it has been reduced to a mere husk of a ritual in the Mass, of Christianity. Most people who like to think of themselves as Christians say Christ never said anything about food, when he in fact made a momentous statement about food; this is, of course, the Last Supper.

During the Last Supper, Christ takes bread, blesses it, and gives it to his disciples saying *"Take this, eat; this is my body"*,[8] and, *"This is my body which is given for you. Do this in remembrance of me"*[9]. He then takes a cup of wine and asks his disciples to drink, referring to the wine as the new covenant in His blood. In the annotations to these verses in the edition of the Bible I am using it says that Jesus Christ transformed a Jewish devotional meal into a continuing association with Himself in death and victory, speaking of His blood is being the mediating reality in the new relationship between God and humanity.

It is noteworthy the foods depicted in this event are the grains and the fruit of the vine, and that Christ, in saying *"do this in remembrance of me,"* is asking of anyone who believes in Him, whenever we are eating a meal we bring Him consciously to mind.

It is extremely significant the foods consumed at the Last Supper were grains and wine. Christ suggests that our main foods should be grains and wine. However I do not think it is wise to drink wine at every meal today simply because the effect of alcohol consumption is to bring about a dimming of consciousness, which is the last thing we need today.

However, if we look at wine as symbolically representing the sap of plants, we can legitimately argue the wine is representative of the vegetable kingdom. Therefore, whole grains are the body of Christ, and vegetables, His blood; in regard to the latter, this idea ties in with the description of assimilation of nourishment being the transformation of food into blood, accompanied with the transmutation of the magnesium of chlorophyll (the essential substance of leafy vegetables) into the iron of the hemoglobin (the essential substance of blood) being critical in this process.

Rudolph Steiner has a great deal to say about Christ, so much so that anything I have read or been taught prior beginning to study his many lecture series on Christ have been exposed as being trite, banal and superficial. One of the most stupendously imaginative descriptions Steiner gives is the key moment in the history of humanity, the Crucifixion. As we know, Christ was crucified, and it was the practice of Roman authorities at that time that a person who is being crucified who was not the worst of criminals would have their agonies and suffering on the cross swiftly cut short by being killed. The method of killing was to insert a spear from the right side of the criminal as he or she hung on the cross and swiftly thrust the spear up under the ribcage towards the left shoulder so as to pierce the heart.

On the particular day Christ was being crucified, the Roman soldiers given this assignment were under the command of a centurion named Longinus. It so happened that in the case of Christ, Longinus wanted to deliver the *coup de grace*. However, he was hard of seeing and he thrust the spear in from the wrong side, thus missing Christ's heart and fulfilling a prophecy.

The key moment of which speak is what happened spiritually when the first drops of the blood of Christ fell on the earth from the wound administered by the spear of Longinus.

Steiner describes this moment by saying if we were in position to perceive spiritually from a vantage point outside the earth, looking down, as it were, on the earth from above, what we would have seen prior to the moment of Christ's blood falling on the earth, is the earth as a spiritual darkness in the spiritual cosmos, a black emptiness or void.

The moment Christ's blood strikes the earth, what had been spiritual darkness, perceived spiritually, then begins to radiate spiritual light throughout the entire spiritual cosmos. From that moment on, Steiner says, the physical earth became Christ's physical body.

Since then, in 1933, Christ has also entered into the etheric realm of the earth, as described in Steiner's lectures series, "*The Re-appearance of Christ in the Etheric*".[10] The etheric realm is, among other things, the realm of the plant kingdom. Pulling all these threads together, we can say eating whole grains and vegetables while consciously bringing Christ to mind means we are entering into a direct relationship with Christ, through His body (the grains) and His blood (leafy greens), but only if we are conscious and aware of this spiritual fact.

If we are not consciously aware of it, as a matter of the course, all kinds of spiritual forces may enter the digestive processes and the assimilating functions, which are not necessary beneficial.

In recent decades the idea the human being can maintain a consciously harmonious relationship with nature and the cosmos has been obliterated. Modern civilization is marked by the tendency to tear the human being out of our relationship with the rhythms of the earth and the cosmos. We now live, at home, school, in the automobile, in the marketplace and at work in a sterile, climate—controlled, hygiene—obsessed environment hermetically cutting us off from the great rhythms of nature and the cosmos.

This lack of understanding and knowledge of the profoundly intimate relationship existing between the human being and the earth and the cosmos has lead to development of a synthetic, artificial lifestyle along with a devitalized, increasingly enfeebled, sickly humanity, and if this trend is not corrected, the prospects for the human population **and the** earth are bleak[11].

The prospects ahead are grim anyway, because it is obvious the various leaders of culture, whatever the cultural institution they happen to be presiding over, are completely at a loss in knowing how to improve the parlous state of the world. The crippled world leadership is amply revealed in all the issues of the day—world wide monetary disorder, food shortages, water shortages, the rapidly increasing cost of living, social unease, an increasingly sick population, with infectious and degenerative illness increasing rapidly; as well as water and air pollution, environmental degradation, to name a few.

This is to be expected, it cannot be otherwise, given the fundamental cause is the way the vast majority of people eats, think, feel and act today. There is no hope in looking for governments, religions, universities, think tanks, and other institutions to guide us out of the present morass, for they, along with each individual, have gotten us into this mess.

Each individual's sickness as revealed by his or her symptomology, indicates he or she is out-of-order, disharmoniously living, eating, thinking and feeling in relation to "the order of the universe" and, therefore, if we wish to change our sicknesses to healthiness, we have to re-order our daily lives in accord with "the order of the universe"[12].

As we move through our processes of healing as a result of eating cooked whole grains and vegetables and doing our ginger compresses over the course of two to three years we'll come to a point we have to widen our daily eating habits to the extent the above statement by George Ohsawa is true for us. That is, whole grains and vegetables will always be our daily staple foods and we widen our daily intake to include in addition any foods we want, including dairy foods, fruit, fish and chicken, chocolate etc. That we can do so is predicated on getting rid of the Chronic Intestinal Stagnation by doing the ginger compress regimen.

What does Chronic Intestinal Stagnation signify? We have feelings, ideas, thoughts, moral qualities of good and evil, hopes, and dreams, desires, attitudes, ambitions, attachments, likes and dislikes etc. It is a grotesque error if we think all these are the results of the totality of physico-chemical activities taking place in our physical body. If we are aware and understand the human being cannot be understood at all as a physical body only, and that in addition to the physical body, we are constituted of etheric body and astral body and "ego", then all that has to do with the spiritual processes enumerated (i.e., feeling, thinking, etc., etc.) are activities of the astral body and "ego". The relationship of these four 'members' of the human being, while we are awake during the day[13], is such that the "ego" is membered to the astral body, which is attached to the etheric body, which permeates the physical body, giving the latter its growth and development, form and function. It is the astral body that is the locus of our attitudes, feelings, thoughts, etc.

Thus, any imbalances and stagnations in the physical body work their way up into the astral body via by the etheric body, and vice versa. As Rudolph Steiner states, "*all disturbances of the physical organism have their origin in the astral body; all disturbances of the astral body have their origin in the physical body*"[14]. It is clear then, if we wish to thoroughly heal ourselves, that our daily eating of whole grains and vegetables is the proper foundation for our healing, but that in itself this is not sufficient for healing to occur. We also need to address the necessity for changing our thinking, feelings, attitudes etc.

Chronic Intestinal Stagnation therefore, represents, imaginatively speaking, nothing less than the physical manifestation of our disturbed astral body, our disturbed soul. It is, so to speak, the dragon of materialism, and the demon of our passions, lusts and desires, uncoiling in our disturbed digestive tract.

Therefore, as we do the regimen of ginger compresses on our abdomen, at the same time changing our diet to whole grains and vegetables and studying yin and yang as well as meditating and self-reflecting, the dissolution of the Chronic Intestinal Stagnation gradually takes place. As a result, we are immeasurably helped in emancipating ourselves of all the habitual, "hand-me-down" concepts, ideas, received prejudices, attitudes and world-views coming from family, church, government, universities.

As we do the ginger compresses along with our daily eating of cooked whole grains and vegetables, the vitality and harmony of intestinal function gradually restores and regenerates itself. As a result, when the time comes for expanding our food choices in addition to cooked whole grains and vegetables, our digestive-metabolic-eliminative functions have no problem in metabolizing and excreting the waste products of these additional foods thoroughly.

NOTES.

1. Rudolph Steiner gives us a very clear indication of this when he says, *"What is contained in the soul of the human being who has passed through the Gate of Death has significance not only for the sphere beyond the earth, but the future earth life itself depends upon what his or her life has been between birth and death. The earth will have the outer configuration that is imparted by the people who have lived upon it. The whole configuration of the planet, as well as the social life of the future, depends on how people have lived in their earlier incarnations. That is the moral element in the ideas of karma and reincarnation"*, Reincarnation and Karma—Their Significance in Modern Culture (Steiner Book Center, 1985, Page 86)
2. I vividly remember the first macrobiotic meal I cooked tasted like sawdust!
3. The word socially is used here to not only include the social and economic ramifications of our daily eating habits, but also the ecological, environmental and spiritual consequences (how we think and behave also affects the spiritual worlds).
4. Three books detailing the disastrous social, economic, and ecological consequences for humanity and the earth of the modern diet are, Culture and Agriculture—*The Unsettling of America* by Wendell Berry, *Diet for a New America* by John Robbins and *The Decline of Beef* by Jeremiah Rifkin.
5. For example, at Pythagoras' Academy, students admitted for spiritual instruction and training were forbidden the eating of beans, as it was thought they were a hindrance to the development of spiritual thinking.
6. The Philosophy Of Oriental Medicine, Part 111: The Macrobiotic Guidebook for Living, George Ohsawa. (Ignoramus Press, 1967, pp 54-56.)
7. Problems of Nutrition—a lecture given in Munich, January 8, 1909. (Anthroposophic Press, 1969, pp.21-22.)
8. Gospel of St. Matthew, Chapter 26, verse 26. The New Oxford Annotated Bible, Revised Standard Version. (Oxford University Press, 1977.)
9. Gospel of St. Luke. Chapter 22, verse 14. (Ibid.)
10. Anthroposophic Press, New York, 1983.
11. The widely accepted idea the earth can exist without being peopled with human beings is symptomatic of the total amnesia existing among today's population regarding the intimate relationship existing between human beings and the earth. If the human population manages to destroy itself there certainly will not be any earth for cockroaches to rule over. For the moment the last human being expires, the physical earth will also expire into the spiritual world.

12. This phrase "the order of the universe" is, granted, a very abstruse and abstract concept but it would take me far beyond the scope and intent of this writing to go into a detailed description of what/whom this "order of the universe" is in reality.

13. In contrast, when we are asleep, the figure lying in the bed is constituted of only the physical and etheric bodies, the astral body and "ego" having left, being tenuously attached with the physical and the etheric body, to enter into a spiritual life in the astral world while our physical body and etheric body are at rest. This is the condition of sleep.

CHAPTER ELEVEN

ON MACROBIOTIC HEALING

The process of healing can also be illuminated as a seven-stage process. First we need to consider the phenomenon of the healing process as being a recapitulation, in reverse, of each individual's process of illness. The diagram, Figure 1., represents this process, called "retracement". The diagram depicts the stages of illness, with, in this example, a person beginning their macrobiotic dietary practice in stage four of the process of illness. He or she begins eating the narrow, delineated cooked whole grains and vegetables program, represented in the diagram band delineated with the yin and yang symbols overlapping to look like the Star of David, (the symbols of yin and yang overlapping one another depict the area of The Spectrum Of Human Food which is balanced with respect to the dynamics of yin and yang of the human organism—whole grains and vegetables (see Figure 1 in Chapter 2).

Speaking imaginatively, the instant we place the first mouthful of cooked whole grains in our mouth, a "mirror" arises out from the ground in front of us, and reflected in it are the stages of illness we have experienced individually, albeit unaware of it, up until that moment. As we continue to eat our macrobiotically oriented dietary program, we experience this "retracement" as a recapitulation, in reverse order, of the stages of illness as we have personally experienced them, each "episode" of illness we previously experienced being relived, in a muted form, and for a shorter period of time.

In Figure 1, a hypothetical example, the "lifeline" represents the passage of a person on a macrobiotic path, which actually begins the day we are born. For it will have occurred to the attentive reader that everyone, whether they realize it consciously or not, is eating, in terms of yin and yang, technically speaking,

---

118

macrobiotically, but most of us are ignorant of this fact, and therefore our eating habits are uninformed, whimsical and conditioned by family and cultural habits and prejudices.

Fig 1.

THE HEALING PROCESS AS "RETRACEMENT".

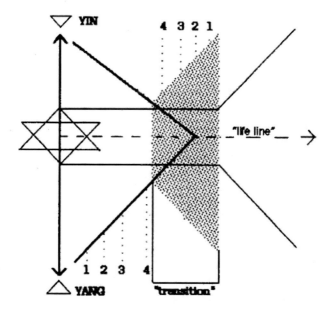

The beginning of the conscious taking of responsibility for our health by adopting a macrobiotic dietary practice begins when the "lifeline" enters the shaded area of the diagram, called the transition period. This is when the "retracement" occurs.

To illustrate what I mean, a man I counseled had started his macrobiotic practice because he had cancer in his left lung. After two years of the restricted diet his lung was free of cancer. Around three years after he started his macrobiotic practice (that is, one year after he was pronounced free of cancer in his lung) he called me one morning in an agitated frame of mind, telling me something "terrible" had happened.

I asked him what was the problem that was so terrible. He had woken up one morning a few days prior to calling me, with the left side of his face paralyzed and he went to the doctor and was informed that he had Bell's Palsy. I first of all reassured him by saying I did not think there is anyway this could be attributed to his macrobiotic dietary program. I then asked him if he had ever experienced this phenomenon of Bell's Palsy before in his life.

He told me that twelve years before he was diagnosed with the cancer he had developed Bell's Palsy. I asked him what had been done about it and he said it had been treated with cortisone and after a few weeks it cleared up. I said the treatment with cortisone had driven the symptoms deeper into his body and they are now resurfacing as part of his healing process and he should not do anything different with his diet and in a few days the Bell's Palsy will disappear. He called me four days later to say the paralysis had gone.

The general rule of thumb is it takes as many months as we are old in years when we start our macrobiotic practice for our body to undergo the major part of the healing process; if we are 35 years old when we begin, it takes 35 months; if we are 56 years old, it takes 56 months, up to the maximum of 84 months or seven years. I therefore recommend we eat the strict, circumscribed macrobiotic dietary practice for at least half this time in months of a person's age in years in the beginning of our macrobiotic life.

Once we have been eating our macrobiotic dietary program for this number of months according to our age when we begin, we are then through the "transition" phase, and it is then time to begin widening our macrobiotic practice to include the additional foods which lie outside the "area of balance", while always maintaining cooked whole grains and vegetables as our daily staple foods.

The maximum length of time it takes for the body to heal itself of the imbalances induced by the standard, modern, conventional diet of meat, eggs, refined sugar, processed food etc., and its associated life patterns, is seven years, as it takes seven years for cells of the human organism to complete a cycle.

From the day we begin our macrobiotic practice, it takes ten days for the blood plasma (the fluid in which the blood cells circulate) to be cleaned out, as it has a 10-day cycle. The white blood cells have a 30-60 day cycle, and the red blood cells a 120-day cycle. From this time on, approximately four months into our macrobiotic dietary practice, the entire bloodstream is renewed and revitalized. Thenceforth the healing process is a mystery yet to be unraveled.

We, as yet, to my knowledge, do not know the details about how the pattern of the healing cycle unfolds in the period between the 120-day cycle of the red blood cells and the seven-year cycle of the whole body. I feel a reasonable hypothesis to suggest is each organ and tissue of the body has its own life cycle, but the length of the cycle in the case, say of liver, large intestine, gall bladder,

I do not know. A possible suggestion is indicated by Rudolf Steiner[1] where he describes some of the organs of the human organism are the manifestations of the same spiritual forces, which manifest as the planets, as follows:

> The spleen is the "Inner Saturn".
> The liver is the "Inner Jupiter".
> The gall bladder is the "Inner Mars".
> The heart is the "Inner Sun".
> The lung is the "Inner Mercury".
> The kidney is the "Inner Venus".

So, it may be reasonable to suggest the cycles of these organs are tied in some way to the cycles of the orbits of these planets with respect to the earth ecliptic, but this will need further research to determine if it is a fruitful line of inquiry. I should note that Steiner did not mention the stomach, small intestine, large intestine or bladder regarding the above idea, only to say the nutritional system and the deposition of substances are expressions of the physical body, in distinction to the etheric and astral bodies.

To my knowledge, as we begin our macrobiotic practice, various bodily events occur, indicating the body is healing itself; although there may well be a cyclical pattern and general order in which the organs heal, my feeling is that each individual undergoes the healing process in his or her own unique way. The pattern of healing of each person expresses itself differently according to the uniqueness of birth date, place of birth, family relationships, diet and upbringing, and a plethora of other aspects of the way a person conducts his or her life including karma and destiny.

Generally speaking, the more acute a condition a person has when beginning their macrobiotic practice, the more dramatic are the expressions of healing experienced, which are referred to as discharges or detoxifications. The more chronic or long-standing the condition, the slower the healing process.

In all instances, unless several factors mitigate against the possibility of healing, the process unfolds in a wave-like fashion, in that we experience peaks and valleys; the peaks when we feel so much better, we have more vitality, calmness, lightness, clarity of mind etc., and the valleys when we feel somewhat run down, lacking in vitality, our appetite is less, we may be experiencing various symptoms like fevers, chills, etc.

There are several factors mitigating against the possibility of healing. This is actually a subject that deserves another book, so I can only be brief and give indications here. The main factor is how much damage has been done to the organism by the taking in of medications, chemicals, radiation, chemotherapy and other poisonous substances. Also, we are not all born equal especially in respect to our physical constitution, which is the expression of the strength of dynamic function of the etheric body, as well as our astral body. How much damage has taken place in our astral body as a result of the way we conduct our lives, not only in this life, but also in previous lifetimes. Thus our karma plays a significant role here.

In addition, our attitude is of deep significance in the healing process or lack of it. If we come to our macrobiotic practice with a sour disposition, looking on a macrobiotic practice as some kind of imposition and deprivation, then our healing process is undermined. I have gone to great length discussing the necessity of changing our way of thinking, and will simply emphasize modern-scientific-materialistic thinking is a fundamentally destructive force which is definitely a major causative factor in the development of degenerative conditions of the body.

The general trend of the healing process is greater improvement in our physical, emotional and psycho-spiritual condition, and as time goes on the peaks and valleys become more and more even, and more widely separated in time until they are rarely experienced. However, it is not to be inferred that we no longer experience healing episodes. The human organism is always healing itself and as time goes on into our second decade and more of our living this way, we may well experience such healing episodes along the way.

In fact, it is a major misunderstanding to think when we are healthy we should never experience periodic episodes of fevers, chills, nasal discharge, aches and pains over the course of time. These episodes are actually very important to experience from time to time, usually at turning points of the seasons, especially Spring and Fall, as they indicate the body is rhythmically adjusting itself to the seasonal rhythm of the year,

Following the dietary practice alone is not sufficient to bring about the experience of true, deep healing, which amounts to a radical self-transformation, such that we are, in profound and subtle ways, not the same person that we were when we started our dietary practice. It must be accompanied by a through-going and persevering re-education of ourselves, working on the psycho-spiritual aspects of healing, which I will address later.

The basics of the superficial symptoms of healing which tend to occur in every one are increased urination, increasing bowel movement and weight loss. Of these, weight loss appears to cause the most consternation, which is ironic and amusing. After all, it is no secret American people tend to be fat to obese, and there are literally dozens of weight loss programs which people use every year (to the tune of spending 4-5 billion dollars per annum) and none of them actually work, except temporarily in some people.

In the case of someone going on a macrobiotic dietary program, which, strictly speaking, is not a diet at all but a daily way of eating based on macrobiotic principles of yin and yang, the general experience is to lose weight, and the weight loss is always beneficial, a sign we are getting rid of a lot of excess toxins stored in dissolving fat deposits.

It sometimes happens that a person gains weight on a strict, circumscribed macrobiotic dietary program, which merely means they needed to gain weight, except in certain circumstances. These are people who have difficulty losing weight on a macrobiotic dietary program. They are, generally-speaking, more likely to be women with what is referred to as a more yang constitution, and did not plan their dietary intake accordingly. Men generally lose weight more easily than women as, internally speaking, men having a more yin constitution than women.

Weight loss can be considerable in a short period of time—I have known people who lost 1-2 lbs. a week. The weight loss will continue until it bottoms out about five pounds under our ideal weight when on a whole grains and vegetable diet, for our height, body type, our level of activity, type of work, etc. After a couple years our weight will come up to our ideal weight, and stabilize there.

In my case I lost 75 pounds, between November 1975 and March 1976, dropping from 195 pounds to 120 pounds (I am five feet, nine and half inches tall), and it increased after two years of eating the strict, circumscribed macrobiotic dietary program, to 125, where it has stabilized over the past 30 plus years.

As to what types of symptoms, in addition to the increases in frequency and amount of urination and bowel movement, and weight loss, we can expect to occur which indicate our body is undergoing the physical healing process, these vary considerably from person to person. However, generally speaking, these "discharges", as they are referred to, can be any one of the following:

> Coughing, sneezing, nasal discharge, fevers and flu—like symptoms, various aches and pains including headaches, as well as fatigue, skin breakouts like pimples and rashes, etc., diarrhea and/or constipation, and in extreme cases vomiting (rarely). In women it is common to experience vaginal discharge and cystitis—type symptoms.

We can, as already discussed, experience emotional "discharges" as part of our healing process also. These are any of the following (you can work out for yourself from what I have already written, which of these emotional discharges are correlated with which organs):

> Anxiety, nervousness, anger, irritability, worry, and depression, sadness, frustration, doubt, loss of confidence, cynicism, and impatience.

—

With regard to the conventional response of anyone experiencing these symptoms, it is to get alarmed because they mean "something is wrong with me", run to the doctor or pharmacy, get the medicine that is "going to making me feel better", and if in fact it does happen to "work", the symptoms indicating the body is healing are suppressed, and therefore the illness is actually driven deeper into the organism. We may feel better eventually, as a result of taking the medication, but fundamentally we are worse off because the illness has not been, fundamentally speaking, addressed at all.

The vast majority of people I have counseled over the years have a medical record as long as your arm, beginning from their childhood. This fact simply testifies to the utter inadequacy of modern scientific medicine, a stark record of its impotency in dealing with illness. However, once we start our macrobiotic way of eating and its concomitant lifestyle, the idea, in this regard, is that we never see another doctor again because we realize the truth that we are the only ones who can take care of ourselves, and if we cannot, we certainly cannot take care of anyone else. Therefore, once we begin our macrobiotic way of life, medical records are a relic of our past.

After all, the major reason why the medical-scientific-pharmaceutical industry has such a firm stranglehold on modern culture is because we have personally abrogated our responsibility for our individual physical, emotional, mental and spiritual well being to the medical profession. In truth, there exists today a co-dependency relationship between the medical system and the population.

It is evident the cost of treating the increasingly sick and diseased population is getting out of control. The notion we have health care is absurd (modern techno-scientific medicine cannot help being utterly impotent and impertinent in respect of offering any solutions to the problem of health, illness and disease). What people want is to get the Federal government to take care of the cost of our personal irresponsibility and ignorance (notwithstanding the cost will be borne by the individual taxpayer anyway). This is not what all the various branches of the illness—treatment industry want, because they do not want the Federal government to control the subsidization of the trillion-dollar industry, as it is now controlled by so-called "health insurance".

Health insurance is totally bogus. What it is is an illness treatment pre-payment plan, for how can paying a monthly premium to some "health-care provider" insure you are going to feel well and vital—it cannot. What you are saying when you buy into a health insurance policy is you have no idea how to take care of your health, so you will put money aside every month to pay for the cost of treating the illness you know you will develop sometime in the future.

When we start our macrobiotic dietary practice and these symptoms of detoxification begin to manifest (no doubt many of the toxins being eliminated are those resulting from the medications, antibiotics, trace element and vitamin supplements we have taken over the years)[2], this means our body is undertaking its healing process. Here I remind you these symptoms also mean our body is healing itself from the regular consumption of meat, eggs, dairy foods, refined, processed, chemicalized foods, alcohol, illicit drugs, etc., and the appropriate response when experiencing them is to let them run their course without interfering with the process.

If we allow these "healing discharges" to run their course then our body's healing forces and immune functions become stronger through doing the work of the detoxification. If we feel it is necessary to do something about the "discharges", there are many, many home remedies we can put together using different combinations of foods in special preparations, using our understanding of yin-yang theory and The Five Transformation Theory. The fundamental principle of home remedies is to support and aid the body during the discharge process, not to stop the processs.[3]

The major question is how do we know when these symptoms of detoxification mean we are, in fact, getting better, or that we are in the throes of a serious illness. That is, are we experiencing a normal healing discharge, or are we in the throes of a serious illness which requires the attention of modern techno-scientific medicine, which is the crisis medicine par excellence, having evolved over the decades dealing with the endless crises arising in us when we have no clue of how to take care of ourselves. Modern techno-scientific medicine has no choice but to adopt a "cut, burn and poison" approach in attempting to put out the symptoms of a person's crisis illness.

Macrobiotic practice, including but not limited to a macrobiotic way of eating cooked whole grains and vegetables every day, is fundamentally a daily practice of becoming better informed of how and why to take care of ourselves, so that we live creatively, developing a healthy body, soul and spirit, insofar as this is possible. What I mean by this is, through karma and destiny it may not be possible for a number of people to thoroughly revitalize and rehabilitate their diseased organism, though I feel that is no reason for not trying. Karma is not to be confused with fatalism since the whole point of karma is we can change it for the better.

I should emphasize that macrobiotic dietary practice and philosophy is far removed from any notion of preventing disease, since this is not possible, nor is it any kind of panacea. I am reminded of a bumper sticker I saw quoting Albert Einstein's *"You cannot both prevent and prepare for war"*. The fact is that to prevent war is to prepare for its inevitability, and so it is with disease. To attempt to prevent disease is to prepare for the inevitable appearance of manifold illnesses. This is amply demonstrated by the abysmal record of modern techno-scientific medicine in the wars it has and continues to conduct against a plethora of illnesses.

There are what I call the four cardinal signs, the presence or absence of which will determine, when we experience these symptoms of detoxification, whether or not we should consider the possibility of availing ourselves of the help of techno-medicine.[4] The four cardinal signs are:

Appetite.
Nausea.
Vitality.
Sleep.

If, when we are experiencing our "discharge symptoms", these four are generally positive, in that our appetite is good, we do not feel sick, our level of vitality is okay, and we sleep well when we go to sleep at night—yes, it is quite normal to have a fever of 104ºF, while bringing up copious amounts of nasal mucus discharge and not feel sick while enjoying a healthy appetite, while our level of vitality is such we can carry out our normal daily routine of going to work etc. I have experienced these many times throughout the three decades of my macrobiotic life. If these four signs are generally positive while we are going through a healing episode (which is what these discharges signify) indicate we are in sound shape, and we will rejoice and be grateful when we experience them, because we know they signify our body is healing itself.

I must repeat myself many times regarding these symptoms. The problem is they have been regarded for hundreds of years by humanity generally as symptoms indicating there is something wrong with our body. In regard of our body, they indicate quite the opposite. What is wrong is our lack of understanding, our ignorance and our prejudices. Our misperceptions of what these bodily symptoms indicate is just one example of many received prejudices ingrained in us by our cultural upbringing of which we have to purge ourselves if we are to have any hope of creating sanity in the world.

Before considering whether we need to go to the doctor or not while we are experiencing symptoms of detoxification, I feel all four signs need to be negative, in that we have no appetite, we feel sick, we are very tired and we have restless sleep. There can be many explanations for why any three of the four may be negative, and yet we are not in any real danger. In any case, anyone starting out on their macrobiotic dietary practice is strongly encouraged to seek out people in their locality who have several years of macrobiotic experience under their belt, who we can talk to if we are unsure of what is happening to us.

All that I have discussed thus far happens unconsciously, in that the body is continuously healing itself as a matter of course. The "wisdom in our body is deeper than our deepest philosophy" to paraphrase the German philosopher Nietzsche, and the spiritual processes undertaken within our body happens unconsciously—we know nothing of the actual processes themselves, other than seeing the results in the symptoms indicating we are experiencing our body detoxifying itself. This is referred to as the mechanical stage of the healing process.

The next stage[6] of the healing process also occurs unconsciously, in that there is a gradual improvement in the sensitivity and acuity of our senses—taste, touch, sight, hearing and smell. According to the Five Transformation Theory the five senses are connected with the condition of the five-paired internal organs of the body as follows:

Hearing—Kidneys/Bladder.
Smell—Lungs/Large Intestine.
Vision—Liver/Gall Bladder.
Taste—Stomach/Spleen-Pancreas.
Touch—Heart/Small Intestine.

Thus, as these organs heal themselves, the senses correlated with them also heal. Also, our sense of direction, orientation in space and time improve and we become more aware of and sensitive to our surroundings, and interested in the events and phenomena happening around us, becoming more attuned and in harmony with the weather, the seasons, the rhythms of the moon and so forth. Our thinking becomes sharper, clearer and more dynamic. This is the **sensory** stage of the healing process.

The next stage is the **emotional** stage, which occurs consciously and unconsciously; that is, in addition to the physical symptoms of detoxification of the body, we also experience emotional symptoms. These I have already described at length in the chapter on the ginger compress. These emotional discharges are usually episodic and short-lived, receding in intensity and extent as the healing of the relevant organs proceeds.

Now, it must not be assumed that once we have healthy organs we will never feel anger, sorrow, frustration, impatience, fear, etc., etc, ever again. These are spiritual realities, which affect our soul life, and, in addition, there are many events and acts taking place in the world today, which are justifiable sources for us to feel angry, sad and worried. I do not need to spell these out for you as you can read about them or see them in the daily news. The question is, how do we react with the anger, sadness or worry we feel? What we need to learn is to acknowledge how we feel and, at the same time, not give vent to them, because if we do we become controlled by our emotions. It is healthy to learn to control our emotions so we can channel the vitality they carry into constructive, positive activities.

If we are willing to face the facts displaying the sickness of our culture as manifested in myriad ways, as, to cite a few examples, gang violence, the "war on drugs", racism, the militia movement, monetary debasement, greed and corruption in government, poisoning of the air, soil and water, despoliation of forests, etc, etc, ad nauseam, we cannot help but feel concerned and worried about the future. However, the way people respond to these problems is to say to themselves, "this is the way things are and there is nothing I can do about it" or to be in denial, or blame these problems on someone or something else, or to protest in various ways running from outright terrorist activities to marching and rallying and asking the government to "do something about it".

However, none of these are going to make one iota of difference to the ongoing course of self-destruction humanity is on until and unless each and everyone of us realize we individually bear the burden of responsibility for creating these problems and issues. Then we can turn to the real task which these symptoms indicate we need to undertake, which is to transform ourselves from being sick, ill, and decrepit human beings to healthy, creative, moral and productive human beings. The beginning crucial step in beginning to heal ourselves is to change our daily way of eating to one based on cooked whole grains and vegetables.

Fear is the one dominant emotion of the times in which we live. There is no question it is the driving force for just about everything people do today. People basically act and live out of fear. The reasons for this lie outside the scope of this book to go into them in any detail. Briefly we are insecure and we are insecure because we do not know what we, as human beings, are. Since we are so mesmerized by materialistic thinking, it is simply unavoidable that we act on our fears and insecurities by seeking to protect ourselves with an assortment of flimsy walls and gates like academic degrees, job security, life-long tenure, pension funds, home ownership, social security, health insurance and so forth. Everyone is enslaved by the delusion that these offer security, whereas they do nothing of the sort.

The truth of the matter is, there is no "safety net" devised which can provide any real security. The only one true safety net is to restore our balance and harmony with the great rhythms of nature and with the spiritual cosmos. This means we must undertake the arduous task of knowing ourselves and our place in creation. And to the degree and extent we are out-of-balance, and dis-eased with respect to nature and the cosmos, to the same degree and extent are we fearful and insecure.

So, looking at people's dietary habits in terms of yin and yang, a dietary intake which has no center, since few, if any, of the foods in the center of the "area-of-balance" in the diagram are being eaten (See Chapter 1, Figure 1), it is inevitable we are being swung back and forth on a wildly oscillating pendulum between extreme yang on the one side, and extreme yin on the other. We thus are perforce running around in our center less existence busily attempting to shore up our lives built on quicksand with all kinds of diversions and dead-ends, like religion, money, sex, politics, alcohol and drugs, power, force, status, insurance policies, etc., etc. In actuality, all these do is increase our insecurity, since there is nothing in them to fill up the emptiness of our rudderless, center less lives, and we become more addicted to these diversions.

If we wish to replace fear and insecurity with confidence and equanimity as we face what the future is going to bring to us, we need to place ourselves on solid ground, physically(eating whole grains and vegetables) and spiritually.

The next stage of the healing process necessarily must take place out of conscious intent—it is only at this **intellectual** stage that we really begin to live our macrobiotic life consciously, since other than the conscious intent of beginning our macrobiotic way of eating, the first stages of healing are unconscious in that we are not aware of what is happening in our bodies other than the appearance of symptoms, as described.

The intellectual stage of healing has to do with consciously changing our way of thinking. I have addressed this issue before but since the problem of thinking is as crucial to our healing as is changing our way of eating, it deserves further discussion. The significance of thinking is pointed out by Rudolf Steiner in the following statement he made in Zurich, November 13, 1917, "*At no other period could it have been said, with regard to the inner necessities of evolution, that clarity of thinking is as essential as eating and drinking are to the maintenance of physical life.*"

As I have stated, the major cause of illness and disharmony afflicting humanity today is scientific materialistic thinking, and this mode of thinking pervades the entire globe. The monumental error of modern scientific materialism is the belief the world is made of nothing but physical matter: that it is constituted of only the phenomena we can count, weigh and measure. This is far from being truthful in conforming to reality. In studying the world of minerals, plants, animals and human beings in attempting to understand how they have come to present themselves to the physical senses, scientific thinking has become analytical and abstract.

It is analytical in that it divides phenomena into smaller and smaller pieces in order to study what underlies the behavior of any object being investigated to try and discover the laws and principles operating in matter. This is perfectly justifiable as long as we understand that any understanding we derive from studying material objects in this way, and what we do learn about the physics and chemical processes tell us nothing about what goes on in living organisms. It is abstract in that in dividing everything up into smaller and smaller pieces for purposes of study and experimentation, isolating and removing them from their natural, normal contexts, we no longer have reality.

Anyone will readily grasp that if we want to study and comprehend the behavioral habits of the polar bear, it would not serve our purposes if we were to relocate the polar bear to the Mojave Desert in order to study it. Yet, modern scientific methodology does something similar every time we put the object of study under a microscope or look at it through a telescope (or any of the modern derivatives of these two instruments); or we place a substance in a test tube or retort and add this chemical or substrate to study its chemical behavior. Rudolf Steiner eloquently states the problem as follows:

> *"Wouldst thou heal man, look into the world on every side, see how on every side the world evolves processes of healing. Wouldst thou know the secrets of the world in the processes of illness and healing, look into the depths of human nature. You can apply this to every aspect of man's being, but you must direct your gaze outwards to the great world of nature and see man in a living relationship to this great world.*

> *People today have become accustomed to something different. They depart from nature as far as possible. They do something which shuts their sight off from nature, for what they wish to examine they lay beneath a glass on a little stand—the eye does not look out into nature, but looks into the glass. Sight itself is cut off from nature. They call this the microscope. In certain connections it might as well be called a nulloscope, for it shuts one off from the great world of nature. People do not know, when something under a glass is magnified, that for spiritual knowledge it is exactly as though the same process were to take place in nature herself. For only think, when you take some minute particle from the human being for the purpose of observation under a microscope, what you then do with this minute fragment is the same as if you were to stretch the man himself and tear him apart. You would be even a worse monster than Procrustes[7] if you were to wrench man and tear him asunder in order to enlarge him as that minute particle is enlarged under the microscope. But do you believe that you would still have the person before you? This would naturally be out of the question. Just as little do you have reality there under the microscope. The truth which has been magnified is no longer the truth, it is an illusory image. We must not depart from nature and imprison our own sight. For other purposes, this can of course be useful, but for a true knowledge of man it is immensely misleading.*

> *Knowledge of man in the true sense must be sought in the way indicated. Starting from the processes of nutrition, it must be followed through to the processes of healing to the processes of human and world education in the widest sense. Or we can put it thus: **from nutrition through healing to civilization and culture.**"* [8](my emphasis).

In order to develop clarity of thought, which is also healthy thinking, we need to realize that outer sense-perceptible phenomena are expressions, manifestations of underlying spiritual realities and forces. The first, most significant step toward undertaking radically changing our thinking is to start eating a macrobiotic way of eating of cooked whole grains and vegetables while we study yin and yang and the Five Transformation Theory as we are learning how to cook macrobiotically.

A casual first impression of yin and yang theory is that it is very straightforward and simple. And it is, but it is also subtle, deeply profound and complex, and it is only through the daily application of yin and yang to our daily nourishment that we can develop the sensitivity, subtlety, vitality and clarity of thought we need. It is important to recognize the understanding of yin and yang, and actually thinking clearly and logically, is dependent, to a much greater degree than people realize, on our internal physical condition. Since it takes, generally speaking, three years of daily macrobiotic practice, consuming a proscribed, limited diet, for the human organism to undergo, so to speak, the bulk of its healing of past dietary excesses and extremes, it takes at least this time of daily study to even begin to understand yin and yang. Furthermore, in order to develop our thinking further so that we understand that thinking is a spiritual activity, I highly recommend studying Rudolf Steiner's volume called **The Philosophy of Spiritual Activity**. This is a difficult book, but the effect of reading it will, in and of itself, bring about a strengthening and enlivening of our thinking abilities.

As we develop our understanding of yin and yang and the Five Transformation Theory, we begin to understand the relationships and interconnections, which is relevant to any line of enquiry we may be undertaking, and our thinking becomes whole and contextual.

This is not the case in today's world. On the contrary, modern, materialistic thinking is fragmented, fragmentary, superficial and illogical, and it cannot help but be so. There are examples everywhere, as can be read in any daily newspaper, journal or magazine; it is a painful experience to read the illogical, abstract and absurd statements printed everyday about any subject not involving mechanical objects like cars and computers, etc.

In the realm of medical science, this type of thinking has reached the depths of absurdity. As a result you will find in this profession specialists of every description imaginable, not only of very organ, system or tissue of the body, but also for different conditions of the same organ, and also different illnesses of the same organ. From modern medical science you would be hard pressed to know the human being is a whole person in which all the organs, tissues, joints, etc., of the body are all interrelated and interconnected to one another, such that imbalances and stagnations in one part of the body affects the conditions of other organs and tissues.

To give just one example, we have in the medical profession ear, nose and throat specialists who study and treat any pathological condition which may develop in them as if they had nothing to do with the rest of the body; therefore, logically, any treatment applied to them which does not take account of their relationships with the rest of the organism are bound to be futile and never-ending. In macrobiotic practice, applying the Five Transformation Theory, it is known the condition of the ear reflects the condition of the kidneys, the nose can reflect the underlying condition of the stomach, heart, upper bronchioles, or the large intestine, and the throat the condition of the kidneys. So, in our daily eating habits, macrobiotically speaking, we consume those foods, which are known to help strengthen the underlying organ condition, and, if necessary, utilize various home cares. Thus, as the condition of the underlying organs improves, so will the condition of the sense organ (ear, nose) or throat related to the relevant organ.

Therefore, since modern scientific thinking is illogical when applied to any domain other than that of material science, leads necessarily to all kinds of errors and absurdities in every domain where modern scientific thinking is applied where it is not pertinent. As a result, today, economists do not understand economics (plainly evident in the current monetary and economic fiasco currently unfolding), politicians have no understanding of politics, educators have no understanding of education, social scientists are at a loss to give cogent analysis of social behavior, modern farmers have no clue about how to husband the land properly, and so forth and so on.

This idea, that we need to take on the responsibility of changing both our way of eating and our way of thinking as described, is absolutely crucial if we are to experience true, deep healing. To change our way of eating without changing way of thinking is like putting new wine into old wineskins; it is fundamentally necessary for us to undertake a rigorous self-training and re-education of our intellect, if we are to have any hope of healing ourselves, and, by extension, the world. And the fact is, it is a lot easier to change our way of eating to cooked whole grains and vegetables, difficult as it may be, than it is to change our way of thinking. To change our way of thinking in the manner indicated is to learn to root out the pervasive, endemic materialistic thinking which has become habitual, to purge ourselves of the conditioned, received "second-hand" thoughts and feelings which have been instilled into us by modern education, family convention, politics, religion and modern media.

As we move on to the next stage of our healing process, the **social** stage, we begin to realize we do not exist in the world merely for our own sakes. We live in a world populated by many people, and as individuals we realize at this stage, our happiness, joy, well being is commensurate with the happiness and well being of all the people living on earth. Conversely, our pain, suffering and hardship is commensurate with that of all the people in the world. In other words, as long as there are people suffering, enduring pain, misery, illness and deprivation of human dignity and happiness, then the wonderful health and vitality we enjoy through the macrobiotic way of eating and changing our way of thinking doesn't really mean a whole lot.

It is plain to see today there is a great deal more suffering, pain, misery, illness and deprivation of human dignity and happiness in the world than there is human joy, happiness, vitality and physical, emotional, mental and spiritual well being.

Social events and activities are the result, the expression of the aggregation of the physical, emotional, mental and spiritual condition of all the people of every culture and society of the world. As we look at society as a whole we become aware of the symptoms of ill individuals, who comprise the vast majority of the population, expressed as social symptoms. Examples of such symptoms of social illness include racism, sexism, the "war on cancer", political and bureaucratic corruption[9] which is endemic today, nuclear weapons development, the "war on terrorism", greed of epic proportions in all elements of society, especially so at the centers of administrative, legislative and judicial branches of government and the military as well as the whole financial industry, homelessness, the national debt, environmental and ecological destruction, etc., etc. These are social symptoms of a profoundly sick culture and are analogous to the symptoms of individual illnesses like AIDS, cancer, diabetes, arthritis, heart disease etc. The world, including nature, so-called "out there", is expressing the physical, emotional, mental, and spiritual disharmony of each individual living today.

As has been well documented all these symptoms of social illness have become more intense, more frequent and more widespread over the past 60 years, such that they are endemic in today's culture. And during the same time degenerative illnesses have become more intense, more frequent and more widespread, as they are also endemic in today's culture. And, coincidentally the modern diet has become more chemicalized, devitalized and industrialized. These are the realities of the world today so it is completely logical to understand we are, each and everyone of us, personally responsible for the present state of the world, which will inevitably relentlessly and more swiftly deteriorate further, unless we each and everyone of use take on personal responsibility for creating a world which is vital, harmonious, creative and peaceful by changing our way of thinking and eating as described in these pages, so that we individually become creative, vital, constructive and peaceful human beings.

This line of thinking throws in obvious relief the utter uselessness and naivety of expecting any solution to the problems we are experiencing to come from the institutions of authority, for they are themselves sick and decrepit. There is no way around it, if we want the world to be a better place to live, we have to change for the better. As Walt Whitman put it *"the human individual is the only fact, and the entrance to all facts"*. Thus we need to look at the facts, let them speak for themselves and respond in the appropriate manner. Today, of course, people are highly indisposed to look at the facts, as they are somewhat inconvenient, and the continuous state of denial will only end when the facts simply overwhelm people.

As of 1984, there were 64 million laws and statutes in the United States (there are probably double that today), and it is plain to see that for all intents and purposes having to do with social stability and progress, they have not made one iota of difference to cultural progress in the intervening 24 years, quite the opposite. The fact is, we cannot legislate morality, truthfulness and honesty, and all laws do is make someone or some group find a way around them, or arrange to have themselves take advantage of the law. Thus laws derived from illogical, absurdly abstract thinking to address the ills of society are analogous to pharmaceutical medications given to sick individuals—they are merely superficial and symptomatic and drive the illnesses of the social organism deeper into the body politic.

Therefore, both because of and in spite of all the many formidable obstacles with which we will have to deal, the most formidable being the head-in-the sand stubborn intransigence of people living in denial of the necessity of changing our daily staple food to cooked whole grains and vegetables and changing our way of thinking in the first instance, at this stage of our healing journey, we resolve to distribute what we know and have experienced through our personal journey of healing in our local community. This we can do in any number of ways, as I have already mentioned.

Another significant factor at this stage of our healing process will become apparent, is we begin to take into account the effect our means of living has on our condition. It is here we need to undertake a rigorous and objective review of the manner in which we earn a livelihood, the lifestyle that goes with it, and its ramifications, ecologically, economically and socially, to see if it is fitting with our macrobiotic practice.

It is the case in many people's lives today, on examining our means of livelihood in this way, we will find we can no longer work at our job or career, if we wish to be comprehensive in our macrobiotic practice, and therefore our healing. There are many examples of jobs and careers today that are thoroughly inconsistent with a healthy, vital, harmonious earthly/cosmic life, and which, if continued while we are undertaking our macrobiotic practice, will definitely undermine our healing process.

In many instances, the realization our job or career is in and of itself contributing to our individual illness, and is counter-productive to ecological, economic and social health puts us in an awkward position. For if it so turns out our assessment is our job or career is contributing to our illness as well as social, ecological and economic illnesses (and if it is doing the former it is certainly doing the latter, and vice-versa), then, if we wish to continue our macrobiotic practice, and we are honest and true to our healing process, we have little choice in giving up our job or career.

In my case, I had been a practicing veterinary surgeon and clinician in large animal practice for three and half years when I adopted my macrobiotic practice. After being on the cooked whole grains and vegetable dietary regimen, as well as studying all the macrobiotic books I could obtain for two and a half more years it did dawn on me my veterinary career was thoroughly incompatible with my macrobiotic practice, Moreover, this glaring inconsistency was making me emotionally, mentally and spiritually ill-at-ease. I was thus confronted with the choice of continuing to tread the path wherever my macrobiotic practice was going to lead me and give up my veterinary career, or quit my macrobiotic practice and continue my career.

Even at this early stage of my macrobiotic practice, I was instinctively, if dimly, aware of the ramifications for the world if more and more people adopted a macrobiotic way of eating as their staple food on a daily basis. It had also become clear to me, through changing my way of eating and studying macrobiotic literature, that modern agribusiness and practices of animal husbandry are the major contributors, not only to the illness of the animals I was seeing every day, but also of the illnesses of people, as well as ecological and economic destruction.

Thus, my choice to resign from the veterinary profession, although as a consequence I experienced a lot of difficulty and pain because of subsequent events in my personal life which resulted from this decision, which I was aware of as possibilities while I pondered my decision for many weeks, was really, in the final analysis, as the saying goes, a no-brainer.

I leave it up to you to work out for yourself whether or not your livelihood is consonant with a sound, healthy macrobiotic life, and consequently, your healing process.

The social level of healing also means we must widen our horizons so as to include in our sense of community the soil and its inhabitants, trees, grasses and plants, insects, birds and animals, rivers and oceans, and the spiritual beings of the spiritual world. Our social environment includes these in addition to the people of the world, and macrobiotic practice is fundamental and essential if there is to be any hope of nature no longer being subjected to forces of destruction entailed in modern scientific thinking and the destructive technology engendered by it.

This means we must change our way of farming and methods of animal husbandry. The farming techniques developed over the past eight decades have gradually wrought greater destruction to the soil, on which the entire world depends for its sustenance. The uses of billions of tons of artificial fertilizer, herbicides, pesticides, and the like have led to the loss of trillions of tons of topsoil. If human beings are going to have a viable future on earth we need to change our farming techniques to those which cease the use of poisonous chemicals as well as help to build a topsoil which is vital, rich and fertile.

The philosophy and practice of agriculture best fitting this purpose is Biodynamic Agriculture, derived from indications given by Rudolf Steiner and pioneered by Eihrenreid Pfeiffer, along with organic farming. This is another subject which is outside the scope of this book, but it cannot be emphasized enough.

Modern culture is at its core anti-life, anti-human and anti-nature. If we wish to have a future, which is creatively, vitally life sustaining the starting point is to change our methods of farming to those of biodynamic and organic farming and start consuming foods grown by these methods.

The next stage of the healing process is the **religious** stage. In order to discuss what religious healing means we first need to clarify the meaning of the word religious. The Oxford English Dictionary states the word is "*of doubtful etymology meaning a life of action or conduct indicating a belief in, reverence for, and desire to please, a divine ruling power in that there is a recognition by man of some higher unseen power as having control over his destiny, and being entitled to obedience, reverence, and worship; the general mental and moral attitude resulting from this recognition, with reference to its effects upon the individual, family, community; and a personal or general acceptance of this feeling as a standard of spiritual and practical life.*"

In his foreword to the I Ching,[10] Carl Jung writes, "*The answering subject (the I Ching) has an interesting notion of itself; it looks upon itself as a vessel in which sacrificial offerings are brought to the gods, ritual food for their nourishment. It conceives of itself as a cult utensil serving to provide nourishment for the unconscious elements or forces (spiritual agencies) that have been projected as gods—in other words to give the attention they need in order to play their part in the life of the individual. Indeed, this is the original meaning of the word "religio"—a careful observation and taking into account of ("religere") the numinous*". In a footnote to this passage Jung states this is the classical etymology; the derivation of religio from religare, "to bind to", came later with the Church Fathers.

Robert Graves, writing in his book, The White Goddess says regarding the word religious: "*the dictionaries give its etymology as "doubtful". Cicero connected it with religere, "to read duly", hence to "pore upon or study divine lore". Some four and a half centuries later, St. Augustine derived it from religare, "to bind back" and supposed it implied a pious obligation to obey divine laws, and this is the sense it has been understood ever since. Augustine's guess, like Cicero's (though Cicero came nearer to the truth), did not take into account the length of the first syllable of the word religio in Lucretius' early "Des Rerum Natura", or the alternative spelling, relligio. Relligio can only be formed from the phrase "rem ligare",—to pick or choose the right thing."*

Rudolf Steiner, in his lecture cycle, "Philosophy, Cosmology, Religion" states religious means the union of man with the divine world; if we are religious in this sense we are clearly conscious of our unification with spiritual agencies,

So, summarizing all these meanings of the word religious means we understand and are clearly conscious of our intimate connectedness and implicit relationships with the spiritual hierarchies, and all the forces, agencies and beings of the spiritual realm; that we know the physical world in all its wondrous, manifold variety of minerals, plants, animals and human beings, is manifesting the actions of the spiritual agencies, and it is our task to study, learn and understand the lore of the gods as revealed in the spiritual and natural laws. And our actions and conduct in our daily lives freely take into account these laws and principles in such a manner that conscientiously, consciously aware of them, we know implicitly how to behave morally and honestly, and so act in any given situation. So when we are presented with problems and difficulties, we know how and when to say and choose to take the right course of action in solving problems and overcoming difficulties.

In conducting this deeply moral religious life we will necessarily feel and increasing sense of reverence, gratitude and devotion to the spiritual agencies we identify as acting on behalf of humanity and the earth.

On the other hand, we will also become aware of those forces, agencies and powers in the spiritual worlds, which are acting to divert, undermine and thwart the progressive spiritual development of the individual. We will be able to identify those forces, which are demonic, and cause people to carry out evil deeds with their evil consequences.

The problem of evil has always been one with which human beings have had to deal if we are to be human at all and the great teachers who have appeared in the course of history have all been religious teachers. However, what these teachers taught so any person applying their instructions to their daily lives so they may become free, independent, courageous, compassionate, moral, healthy, joyful, vital and creative has degenerated over the course of time into religions. The mark of religions today is they have become mere husks of empty ritual, people going through the motions of what it means to be religious, the teachings reduced to creeds, codes, and empty rhetoric, for the institutions of the religions have become all important, not the teaching which originated the institution. They have indeed become worldly, secular centers of power, authoritarian, rife with hypocrisy and cant, and far removed from being in any sense of the term, religious.

From my perspective, it is easy to see it is the individuals who least understood the teachings which they profess who founded the institutions, and over time the institutions takes on the characteristics of a lower life form which has to be continually fed so as to continue to exist while it seeks to fill the world with copies of itself. Thus the organism needs to be continually fed so as to exist, and all these people become so consumed with feeding the organism they forget what the teachings are about in the first place, and, moreover, fail to develop them so they fit the times in which they operate.

As St. Paul wrote, "*the letter killeth, it is the spirit which giveth life*". Since the spirit has long since fled the premises, what has become sacred to these institutions is the letter of the law, the codifications, the rigid stratification of hierarchy, the exclusion of anyone who refuses to be constrained by these limitations on what it means to be a human being. As soon as anyone comes along and declares something perceived by them a threat to their naked authoritarianism and worldly ambitions, they are declared a heretic and burnt at the stake, either literally or figuratively.

It is evident then, if we wish to heal ourselves we need to purge ourselves of the psychic dross of tired, worn-out, habitual empty phrases, and second-hand hollow rhetoric promulgated by all the religions of the world. That is to say, we need to quit merely belonging to religions and start living religious lives in our every day life. Everyone has direct access to the spiritual world, ("*seek and ye shall find, ask and ye shall be answered, knock and the door will be opened*") no one needs an intermediary, so why belong to a religion when the original intent of all the great original, authentic teachers is to teach us how to be free?

The final stage of the healing process is spiritual healing. As I mentioned in another context, all these stages of healing need to be recognized as being built up one on top of the other, so as we go through each stage we retain each of the previous stages so that they are all being undertaken concurrently and conterminously.

This stage of the healing process is a subject of such proportion I am not even going to attempt to try and do it justice. In essence, what it consists of is not only being aware and conscious of the spiritual fact we are intimately bound up with and interrelated to a vast hierarchy of spiritual beings and agencies, it is here we take the steps to get to know how to perceive and communicate with these spiritual beings, to become familiar with them by name and activity, etc. As this is a very difficult process to describe and undertake and the instructions and knowledge of how this can be accomplished are already presented in the voluminous work of Rudolf Steiner. I thus recommend the reader who wishes to go deeper into this stage of the healing process to read and study the books by Steiner I have listed in the bibliography as a place to start our individual process of learning to perceive, know and communicate with, in a state of wide-awake consciousness, while in the physical body, the spiritual worlds and the beings which populate it.

NOTES.

1. In his lecture cycle *Occult Physiology* (Anthroposophic Press).
2. The population of the US is 5% of the world population and consumes more than 60% of world sales of pharmaceutical medications, approximately 64 billion dollars per year. See the article "Time's Up" in the Wall Street Journal, August 12, 1997.
3. Two useful publications to consult on home cares are *Macrobiotic Home Remedies* by Michio Kushi (Japan Publications, 1985) and *Natural Healing from Head to Toe* by Herman and Cornellia Aihara (Avery Publishing Group, 1994)
4. Of course, many people begin a macrobiotic practice without having access to or even trying to contact people with long-time experience of macrobiotic practice. Thus, unfortunately, when they begin to experience these detoxifications symptoms conclude they are getting worse, and blame the macrobiotic dietary regimen they have adopted. Well, they are correct in that the macrobiotic dietary regimen is responsible for their body cleansing, but wrong in thinking their condition is getting worse! In these instances people generally abandon the dietary regimen altogether and go back to a familiar diet.
5. The reason we do not have all the vitality in the world at this time is due to our body using its inner vitality of healing to initiate and carry through the detoxification process, so we do not necessarily have much vitality ourselves. Rest assured, though, once the detoxification process has run its course, we feel more vitality than we have in a long time.
6. In referring to the stages of healing/illness, I do not mean to say all the stages are clearly demarcated one from the other in actual experience. The way to read these descriptions of the stages is they are a way of seeing the way the process unfolds. In actuality, a person may be experiencing symptoms of two or three stages at the same time.
7. Procrustes is a character in classic Greek Mythology. He was a robber who stretched or amputated the limbs of travelers to make them conform to the length of his bed. He was killed by Theseus.
8. In *Man as Symphony of The Creative Word* (Rudolf Steiner Press, London, 1970, pp. 188-189).
9. Lord Acton made the famous statement, "*Power corrupts and absolute power corrupts absolutely*". If this statement is correct, then its corollary, "the corrupt seek power and the absolutely corrupt seek absolute power" is also correct.
10. *I Ching or Book of Changes*, the Richard Wilhelm translation, translated into English by Cary Baynes, Third Edition (RKP, 1974, p xxviii).

CHAPTER TWELVE

GETTING STARTED

This chapter is for those readers who wish to get going as soon as possible. Before going into suggestions on what you need to buy one important question always comes up, which is the question of daily water/liquid intake. A widespread misconception is the daily liquid intake of people eating macrobiotically is insufficient. This may seem true to those eating the standard American fare of meat and sugar, potatoes, sugar, etc., along with numerous chemicals in the form of additives, vitamins and medications as well as refined salt. This is a daily fare that will generally cause dehydration, so the natural response is excessive thirst.

The kidneys are filtering organs, not, as is commonly supposed, a flushing organ (a function performed by the bladder), and they have a limited capacity of fluid they can filter in any given unit of time. The consumption of excessive amounts of liquid thus puts a burden on the kidneys and they begin to get tired out over the course of time, and they become weak, with the result that the last I looked there are 1 million cases of kidney failure per year in the US, and weakened kidneys also lead to mineral depletion.

Macrobiotic foods are 75-90% water after they have been cooked. Thus we get plenty of liquid in the food. It is recommended if we are eating macrobiotically to consume 3-5 eight ounces glasses of liquid a day, which includes teas as well as water (this does not include the one bowl of miso soup we eat a day). After that, drink only when thirsty.

Another point is if we sweat excessively, this means we are drinking too much liquid. The commonly held view is we need to drink more to replace the fluids we lose through copious sweating, which actually only compounds the problem.

140

If we find we are urinating more than three to five times daily this means we are consuming too much liquid. If we need to urinate at night after retiring we can be sure we have kidney/bladder weakness, also called "water disease".

The Alchemycal Pages.

This is my website which is a companion to this book, and vice-versa. There is a tremendous amount of additional information there and you will find it very helpful. The URL is: http//www.alchemycalpages.com

For additional macrobiotic resources on the internet, just type the word macrobiotic into your search engine.

A Shopping List.

> 25 lbs organic short grain brown rice.
> 5lbs organic millet.
> 5lbs rolled oats.
> 2 lbs organic aduki beans.
> 1 lb organic unpasteurized 2 1/2 year old or older Barley Miso.
> 8 ounces of organic Umeboshi Plums.
> 1 pkt. pickled daikon root or 1 jar organic sauerkraut, plain.
> I lb Si-salt.
> I liter virgin organic olive oil or sesame oil.
> I bottle of organic shoyu or tamari soy sauce.
> I 16 oz bottle of Rice Syrup.
> 4-6 ounces of kombu or wakame sea vegetable.
> I lb organic brown unhulled sesame seeds.
> 8 ozs Kudzu.
> *Self-Healing Cookbook* by Kristina Turner and/or *Basic Macrobiotic Cooking* by Julia Ferre.
> A 2-3 liter stainless steel pressure cooker (although this is not mandatory). Pressure-cooked grains offer significant improvements over boiling them. Also beans are easier to cook in a pressure cooker.)

All this will set you back about $120-$150 without the pressure cooker (which costs between $100-$150 depending on the brand.). However, most of the items in the list will take anywhere from a week to 10 weeks to consume, so although the initial outlay is significant, in the long run eating macrobiotically is significantly more economical than the standard fare (probably 30-50% more economical). Of course, the pressure cooker will last generations.

Organic or bio-dynamically grown vegetables can be purchased every couple days or so.

Food Resources.

Please support your local natural food store, if you have one, whenever possible. If there is a farmer's market near you, obtain vegetables there. There are a number of macrobiotic mail order companies if you happen to live in an area where some items are hard to find—use the internet to search for these. Also, if practically feasible for you, start growing vegetables in your backyard.

Final Remarks.

Although I have mentioned it at various junctures throughout the book, I must make myself perfectly clear. The information provided in this book is to encourage and support you in considering a macrobiotic approach to any health problems as well as to maintain your health, along with home remedies (especially the Ginger Compress and the Daikon Bath) as the most natural and gentle way to help your body heal itself.

The information is given with the caution that if you decide to do so, you take full responsibility for so doing, according to the guidelines, based upon your interpretation, understanding and practice. Although in many instances the human body's response to a macrobiotic dietary practice is to resolve most if not all of your symptoms, no guarantees are given that they in fact will.

Furthermore, the disappearance of chronic illness symptoms does not mean the causes have disappeared or that a cure has been effected. It takes many years of diligent application, study, self-reflection and practice to see a resolution of symptoms of imbalance, some of which are resulting from 10, 20, 30 or more years of living an out-of-balance way of living.

It is the individual's responsibility to work through the ups and downs of the healing process and to keep learning from everything that occurs, and to keep studying. Your decisions are solely yours and are in fact the only valid decisions. Thus, the information contained in this book is not, nor is it intended to be, medical advice. If you desire medical advice for your condition, please contact the appropriate medical professional.

BIBLIOGRAPHY

All the books listed here have been instrumental in informing the writing of *The End Of Medicine*, and are complementary to it. I highly recommend they are obtained and studied.

Rudolf Steiner
Theosophy
An Outline of Occult Science.
Knowledge of Higher Worlds.
Christianity as a Mystical Fact.
The Philosophy of Spiritual Activity.
Man as Symphony of The Creative Word (Rudolf Steiner Press).
Occult Physiology.
Karmic Relationships, Vol. 1-VIII. (Rudolf Steiner Press).
Reincarnation and Karma—Their Significance in Modern Culture.
(Unless otherwise stated, all titles published by Anthroposophical Press).

Authorized King James version of The Bible.

George Ohsawa.
The Philosophy of Oriental Medicine.
Zen Macrobiotics.
Guidebook for Living.
Jack and Miti in The West.
Acupuncture and The Philosophy of The Far East.
(All titles published by The George Ohsawa Macrobiotic Foundation.).

Noboru Muramoto.
Healing Ourselves.
(Avon Publications, 1972).

—

Richard Wilhelm & Cary Baynes (Translators).
I Ching or Book of Changes.
(RKP, 1974}.
Lao Tzu Tao Te Ching.
(Tr Gia-Fu Feng and Jane English, Harper &
Row, 1972).
Chuang Tzu Inner Chapters.
(Tr Gia-Fu Feng and Jane English, Harper &
Row, 1972).
Basic Writings, (tr. Burton Watson, Columbia
University Press, 1964.)
Dr. Morishita MD Overcoming Cancer—The Natural Medicine
Diet Therapy,
(Living Naturally Center, Los Angeles, 1998,)
Michio Kushi Your Face Never Lies.
(Avery Publications, 1983.)
Natural Healing Through Macrobiotics.
Oriental Diagnosis—How To See Your Health.
Macrobiotic Home Remedies.
(All Published by Japan Publications.)
Theodore Andre Cook The Curves Of Life,
(Dover, 1979).
Dr. Gerhardt Schmidt MD
The Dynamics of Nutrition.
The Essentials of Nutrition.
(Biodynamic Literature).
Wendell Berry Culture and Agriculture—The Unsettling of
America.
(Avon, 1978).
Herman Aihara Basic Macrobiotics.
(Japan Publications).
Herman & Cornellia Aihara
Healing from Head to Toe—Traditional
Macrobiotic Remedies.
(Avery Publishing).
Anonymous Meditations on The Tarot—A Journey into
Christian Hermeticism.
(Amity House)
Quest for The Holy Grail.
(Penguin Books)
Kristine Turner Self-Healing Cookbook.

	(Earthtones Press.).
Anne Marie Colbin	Food and Healing.
	(Vintage Books).
Rudolf Valentine MD	Diet and Nutrition—A Holistic Approach.
	(Himalayan Institute Press.).
Ralph Waldo Emerson	Essays and Lectures.
	(The Library of America.).
Plato	The Collected Dialogues.
	(Princeton University Press).
Carl Ferre	The Pocket Guide to Macrobiotics.
	(The Crossing Press.)
Julia Ferre	Basic Macrobiotic Cooking.
	(George Ohsawa Macrobiotic Foundation.)

Medard Gabel with The World Game Laboratory

Ho-ping: Food For Everyone—Strategies to Eliminate Hunger on Spaceship Earth. (Anchor Books—1979.)

Lady Evelyn Barbara Balfour

The Living Soil and The Haughey Experiment. (Devin-Adair Co; Revised edition, 1950)

LaVergne, TN USA
19 November 2009
164702LV00007B/198/P